Colon Polypectomy

Antonio Facciorusso · Nicola Muscatiello
Editors

Colon Polypectomy

Current Techniques and Novel Perspectives

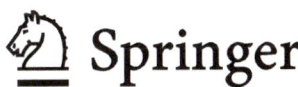 Springer

Editors
Antonio Facciorusso
Gastroenterology Unit, Department
of Medical Sciences
University of Foggia
Foggia, Italy

Nicola Muscatiello
Gastroenterology Unit, Department
of Medical Sciences
University of Foggia
Foggia, Italy

ISBN 978-3-319-59456-9   ISBN 978-3-319-59457-6   (eBook)
https://doi.org/10.1007/978-3-319-59457-6

Library of Congress Control Number: 2017960824

Printed on acid-free paper

This Springer imprint is published by Springer Nature
The registered company is Springer International Publishing AG
The registered company address is: Gewerbestrasse 11, 6330 Cham, Switzerland

To our Director-General Antonio Pedota and our Medical Director Laura Moffa for their continuous and enthusiastic support

The greatest good you can do for another is not just to share your riches but to reveal to him his own.

– Benjamin Disraeli

Preface

Since its introduction in clinical practice in the early 1970s, colon polypectomy has become a standard procedure for treating noninvasive mucosal adenomas and neoplasms, with the aim to interrupt the adenoma-carcinoma sequence leading to invasive cancer.

However, despite proven effectiveness, polypectomy techniques are often heterogeneous and lack complete standardization, particularly in some aspects such as submucosal injection solutions or resection methods.

Proper removal of polyp needs not only technical skill but also complete and updated knowledge of endoscopic equipment and awareness of potential complications according to morphology and size of the mucosal lesion.

In the colorectal cancer screening era, detection and resection of all polypoid lesions are the main goals of quality colonoscopy, and submitting all resected polyps to pathologic examination still represents the standard of care.

Furthermore, other important aspects play a fundamental role in this setting, particularly increasing adenoma detection rate during screening colonoscopy and scheduling a proper surveillance program according to polyp features. Finally, the endoscopist should take into account other patient-related characteristics which may increase the risk of complications, such as ongoing therapy with antithrombotic agents or concomitant systemic disease.

For these reasons, it seemed rational to produce a book that represents much of the current evidence and controversies on colon polypectomy. In order to overcome bias related to a single-center experience, outstanding experts from all over the world have been invited to contribute to this project.

This is an exciting time to be in the field of endoscopy as so many changes are simultaneously occurring at multiple levels of our understanding, and there is an increasing interest toward new techniques which have been recently developed.

We are confident our book will be of interest either to the expert endoscopist who wants to stay abreast with the novel advancements in the field or to the trainees who will likely benefit from authors' experience to improve their skills.

Foggia, Italy   Antonio Facciorusso
July 2017   Nicola Muscatiello

Contents

Contributors

Matteo Antonino Gastroenterology Unit, University of Foggia, Foggia, Italy

Maria Antonia Bianco Gastrointestinal Unit, ASL Na3 SUD, Torre del Greco, Naples, Italy

Antonella Bonitatibus Department of Medicine and Ageing Sciences, "G. D'Annunzio" University, Chieti, Italy

Cristina Bucci Gastrointestinal Unit, ASL Na3 SUD, Torre del Greco, Naples, Italy

Rosario Vincenzo Buccino Gastroenterology Unit, University of Foggia, Foggia, Italy

Renato Cannizzaro Gastroenterology Unit, Centro di Riferimento Oncologico, IRCC, Aviano, Italy

Vincenzo Canzonieri Pathology Unit, Centro di Riferimento Oncologico, IRCCS, Aviano, Italy

Valentina Del Prete Gastroenterology Unit, University of Foggia, Foggia, Italy

Konstantinos Efthymakis Department of Medicine and Ageing Sciences, "G. D'Annunzio" University, Chieti, Italy

Antonio Facciorusso Gastroenterology Unit, University of Foggia, Foggia, Italy

Cesare Formisano Department of Clinical Medicine and Surgery, Surgical Digestive Endoscopy Unit, University of Naples Federico II – School of Medicine, Naples, Italy

Mara Fornasarig Gastroenterology Unit, Centro di Riferimento Oncologico, IRCCS, Aviano, Italy

Giuseppe Galloro Department of Clinical Medicine and Surgery, Surgical Digestive Endoscopy Unit, University of Naples Federico II – School of Medicine, Naples, Italy

Federico Iacopini Gastroenterology Endoscopy Unit, S. Giuseppe Hospital, Albano L., Rome, Italy

Tonya Kaltenbach San Francisco Veterans Affairs Medical Center, San FranciscoCA, USA

Francesco Laterza Department of Medicine and Ageing Sciences, "G. D'Annunzio" University, Chieti, Italy

Raffaella Magris Gastroenterology Unit, Centro di Riferimento Oncologico, IRCCS, Aviano, Italy

Stefania Maiero Gastroenterology Unit, Centro di Riferimento Oncologico, IRCCS, Aviano, Italy

Angelo Milano Department of Medicine and Ageing Sciences, "G. D'Annunzio" University, Chieti, Italy

Fabio Monica Division of Gastroenterology and Digestive Endoscopy, Azienda Sanitaria Universitaria Integrata di Trieste, Academic Hospital Cattinara, Trieste, Italy

Nicola Muscatiello Gastroenterology Unit, University of Foggia, Foggia, Italy

Matteo Neri Department of Medicine and Ageing Sciences, "G. D'Annunzio" University, Chieti, Italy

Vasilios Papadopoulos Hepatogastroenterology Unit, National and Kapodistrian University, Attikon University General Hospital, Athens, Greece

Giulia Maria Pecoraro Division of Gastroenterology and Digestive Endoscopy, Azienda Sanitaria Universitaria Integrata di Trieste, Academic Hospital Cattinara, Trieste, Italy

Simona Ruggiero Department of Clinical Medicine and Surgery, Surgical Digestive Endoscopy Unit, University of Naples Federico II – School of Medicine, Naples, Italy

Teresa Russo Department of Clinical Medicine and Surgery, Surgical Digestive Endoscopy Unit, University of Naples Federico II – School of Medicine, Naples, Italy

Yutaka Saito Endoscopy Division, National Cancer Center Hospital, Tokyo, Japan

Roy Soetikno San Francisco Veterans Affairs Medical Center, San Francisco, CA, USA

Donato Alessandro Telesca Department of Clinical Medicine and Surgery, Surgical Digestive Endoscopy Unit, University of Naples Federico II – School of Medicine, Naples, Italy

Konstantinos Triantafyllou Hepatogastroenterology Unit, National and Kapodistrian University, Attikon University General Hospital, Athens, Greece

Jessica X. Yu Division of Gastroenterology and Hepatology, Stanford University School of Medicine, Stanford, CA, USA

Fabiana Zingone Gastrointestinal Unit, ASL Na3 SUD, Torre del Greco, Naples, Italy

Classification of Colon Polyps and Risk of Neoplastic Progression

Renato Cannizzaro, Raffaella Magris, Stefania Maiero, Mara Fornasarig, and Vincenzo Canzonieri

1.1 Introduction

Intestinal polyps are projections from the mucosal surface that bulge into the visceral lumen and they are classified on the basis of their clinico-pathological qualities (i.e., neoplastic versus non-neoplastic) (Table 1.1) and/or their histopathological characteristics (Table 1.2). Adenomas are recognized as the precursor lesions for colorectal carcinoma [1]. Endoscopically, any superficial intestinal lesion may be described as follows: polypoid type (pedunculated, sessile, semi-pedunculated lesions), non-polypoid type (slightly elevated, flat, slightly depressed lesions) [2, 3].

Table 1.1 Clinico-pathological classification of polyps

Neoplastic mucosal polyps
Benign (adenoma)
Tubular adenoma
Tubulovillous adenoma
Villous adenoma
Malignant (carcinoma)
Noninvasive carcinoma
Carcinoma in situ
Intramucosal carcinoma
Invasive carcinoma (through muscularis mucosae)
Non-neoplastic mucosal polyps
Hyperplastic polyp (including serrated polyps)
Mucosal polyp (normal mucosa in a polypoid configuration)
Juvenile polyp (retention polyp)
Peutz–Jeghers polyp
Inflammatory polyp

R. Cannizzaro (✉) • R. Magris • S. Maiero • M. Fornasarig
SOC Gastroenterologia Oncologica, Centro di Riferimento Oncologico, IRCCS, Aviano, Italy
e-mail: rcannizzaro@cro.it

V. Canzonieri
SOC Anatomia Patologica, Centro di Riferimento Oncologico, IRCCS, Aviano, Italy

© Springer International Publishing AG 2018
A. Facciorusso, N. Muscatiello (eds.), *Colon Polypectomy*,
https://doi.org/10.1007/978-3-319-59457-6_1

Table 1.2 Histopathological classification of polyps

Epithelial
Conventional adenoma
Tubular adenoma
Tubulovillous adenoma
Villous adenoma
Flat adenoma
Serrated polyps
Hyperplastic
Sessile serrated adenoma
Mixed polyps
Traditional serrated adenoma
Polypoid adenocarcinoma
Inflammatory
Mucosal prolapse-associated polyps
Inflammatory pseudo-polyp
Polypoid granulation tissue
Infection associated polyp
Hamartomatous
Peutz–Jeghers polyp
Juvenile polyp
Cowden syndrome
Cronkite Canada syndrome
Stromal
Inflammatory fibroid polyp
Fibroblastic polyp
Schwann cell neurilemmoma
Ganglioneuroma
Leiomyoma
Lipoma
Lipohyperplasia of ileo-cecal valve
Gastrointestinal stromal tumor
Neurofibroma
Granular cell tumor
Lymphoid
Prominent lymphoid follicle
Lymphomatous polyposis
Endocrine
Differentiated endocrine tumor
Other
Prominent mucosal fold
Everted appendiceal stump
Elastotic polyp
Endometriosis
Mucosa xanthoma
Melanoma/clear cell sarcoma
Metastasis
Malignant (carcinoma)
Noninvasive carcinoma
    Carcinoma in situ
    Intramucosal carcinoma
Invasive carcinoma (through muscularis mucosae)
Non-neoplastic mucosal polyps
Hyperplastic polyp (including serrated polyps)
Mucosal polyp (normal mucosa in a polypoid configuration)
Juvenile polyp (retention polyp)
Peutz–Jeghers polyp
Inflammatory polyp

Recently, it has been recognized that some hyperplastic lesions, with serrated morphology, can exhibit a significant risk of neoplastic progression, through the so-called serrated pathway [1].

1.2   Histological features of adenoma

1.2.1   Adenoma

Adenomatous polyps contain epithelial neoplasia account for approximately 10% of polyps [2, 4].

From a histological point of view, three types of adenomas are defined: tubular adenomas, villous adenomas, tubulovillous adenomas depending on their predominant glandular pattern [5]. The difference between tubular and tubulovillous adenomas depends on the percentage of volume of adenoma that is villous (20% in tubulovillous, 80% in villous) [2]. Tubular adenomas are small and present mild dysplasia whereas large adenomas often exhibit villous architecture and are associated with more severe degree of dysplasia [5]. The highest morbidity and mortality rates are associated with villous adenomas.

1.3   Adenoma Size

Adenomas can be classified by size in three classes: diminutive (1–5 mm diameter); small [6, 9], to and large (more than 10 mm) [4]. Size and histology of adenomas correlate with the risk of progression to carcinoma.

Adenomas of 10 mm of diameter or more are considered advanced, instead adenomas which are less than 1 cm are considered advanced when contain more at least 25% villous features, high grade dysplasia or carcinoma [4]. Diminutive polyps are commonly encountered during endoscopy and less than 1% of them are villous or contain a focus of high grade dysplasia.

1.4   Adenoma Carcinoma Sequence

Molecular studies have reported that several signaling pathways are involved in the carcinogenesis of Colorectal Cancer (CRC) [6, 7]. Molecular complexity can explain the morphological heterogeneity of CRC, in terms of site, grade, and type of the tumor [6, 8, 9]. Studies have centered on genetic changes of the three main categories of genes: (1) Tumor suppressor genes (TSG), such as APC, DCC, TP53, SMAD2, SMAD4, and p16INK4α; (2) protooncogenes, such as K-ras, N-ras, and (3) DNA repair genes, such as MMR and MUTYH [10–12]. The first elucidated is suppressor or chromosomal instability, the classical pathway recognized in the Fearon and Vogelstein genetic model [6, 10, 13]. It includes FAP tumors and 80% of sporadic colorectal carcinomas. This model proposes that mutations in concrete genes, in particular TSGs, cause the histopathological sequence of the progression of CRC [10]. Changes start with the mutation or loss of APC gene, followed by

KRAS mutations, TP53 and DCC mutations [10]. 70–80% of colorectal tumors present APC gene mutations, instead K-ras mutations are found in 40% of tumors [10, 14–16]. The Fearon–Vogelstein model is even now considered valid for illustrating the concept of multiple steps of tumor progression. The sequences of proposed changes are the result of a statistical analysis so not all individuals have to show all of the changes [10].

The second elucidated pathway is the mutating or microsatellite instability (MIN) pathway that is responsible for the development of hypermutating carcinomas [6]. It includes the Lynch syndrome tumors and approximately 15% of sporadic tumors [10]. Lynch syndrome is caused by a mutation in one of the genes encoding proteins involved in mismatch repair (MMR) [6, 17]. Mutation on MMR genes provoke genomic instability that leads to hypermutator phenotype known as microsatellite instability determining an accelerated progression to carcinoma [10, 18].

The third, alternative, mechanism of carcinogenesis has been described as an epigenetic process. A frequently encountered mechanism responsible for silencing of TSGs is the hypermethylation of gene promoter associated CpG Island (CIMP), involved in the regulation of transcription [6, 19]. These epigenetic changes create instability in the genes as a result of the inactivation of TGS or MSI or CIN repair genes. The causes that activate the hypermethylation process are not clear. Environmental factors that could be involved are lesion due to chemotherapeutic agents, the ingestion of folates but the reasons or genetics that regulate this phenomenon are not well known [10, 20].

1.5   Serrated Lesions

Serrated polyps are defined as epithelial lesions with a serrated or "saw-toothed appearance" on histologic section due to infolding of crypt epithelium [21]. Serrated lesions vary from hyperplastic polyps (HP), sessile serrated adenomas (SSAs), dysplastic serrated polyps (traditional serrated polyps), or mixed lesion/polyps [2, 21].

1.5.1   Hyperplastic Polyps

HPs are highly prevalent diminutive sessile polyps that occur in the distal part of the colon and rectum. HPs are also the most frequent serrated polyps (80–90%) and they represent the 29–40% of all the polyps [22]. They usually have a diameter less than 5 mm and microscopically they exhibit distinct surface patterns. They show elongated crypts with serrated architecture in the upper half part of crypts or sometimes in the upper third and on the surface of the crypts leading to an irregular distension and a serration in the upper half of crypts [1, 21]. These surface patterns correspond to the histological subtypes: microvesicular serrated polyps (MVSPs), goblet cell serrated polyps (GCSPs), and mucin poor type (very rare) [1, 21]. Nuclei, in cells of the basal part are small, uniform, and basally oriented and nuclei in the upper part of the crypts are not crowed and there is no hyperchromasia [1, 2].

There is no cytologic dysplasia or intraepithelial neoplasia, no structural or architectural changes [1]. The two different histological subtypes differ also in molecular profiles. MVSPs show BRAF mutation and an increased level of susceptibility to aberrant methylation at promoter regions. GCSPs show KRAS mutation which is not shown in SSAs but there is some evidence that large GCSPs can progress to SSAs. So classifying HPs has no clinical importance [21].

Recently, it has been discovered that HPs could possess some malignant potential in the setting of hyperplasic polyposis syndrome. Patients presenting hyperplastic polyposis syndrome present: five or more serrated polyps proximal to the sigmoid colon with two or more larger than 10 mm in diameter; a total of more than 20 polyps, or a serrated polyp proximal to the sigmoid colon and a first-degree relative with the syndrome [23, 24]. The risk of malignant progression for most of the small distally located HPs in the colorectum is very low [1]. Polyps larger than 10 mm, instead, should be removed because some studies demonstrated that they could have malignant potential [1].

1.5.2 Sessile Serrated Adenomas

Sessile serrated polyps are heterogeneous lesions usually found in proximal colon (75%). They are less common than HP and have been suggested to account around 15–25% of all serrated polyps and 1.7–9% of all polyps [22]. SSAs are characterized by hyperserrations with rectangular dilatation of the whole crypts with or without the presence of mucus, T and L branching at the crypt base, and pseudoinvasion into the mucosal layer. Distortion in the bases of the colonic crypts is often present with an increased number of goblet cells, slightly enlarged vesicular nuclei with prominent nucleoli, and proliferation zone in the middle third of the crypts [1, 2, 4].

SSAs often produce excessive extracellular mucin, and stain positively for MUC5AC and MUC2 which are present in the surface of the polyp [22].

Endoscopically, SSAs appear as flat, sessile, or slightly elevated lesions, malleable, and often covered by a thin layer of yellowish mucus and usually they are larger than 5 mm in diameter [1, 21].

Their surface is generally smooth or granular and often their borders are irregular and poorly defined [21].

SSAs have two defining molecular genetic characteristics that indicate their relationship to MVSPs and to sporadic colon rectal cancer with high levels of microsatellite instability (MSI-H), namely BRAF-mut and high levels of CpG island methylation [21, 25, 26]. However, some contradictory studies highlight that they differ for anatomical distribution.

1.5.3 Dysplastic Serrated Polyps

Dysplastic serrated polyps are less common than conventional adenomas or HP, accounting for only 1–2% of all polyps [21]. Dysplastic serrated polyps show neoplastic crypts with serrated structures [2].

They share histological features as serrated gland component and the presence of eosinophilic dysplastic epithelium [2, 21]. Dysplastic serrated polyps can also be divided into two categories: SSA with dysplasia (SSAD) and traditional serrated adenoma (TSA). SSADs exhibit inverted T L shaped crypt bases, crypt branching and dilatation, presence of mature goblet cells in the crypt base or they show SSA characteristic next to an area of serrated or conventional dysplasia [21]. TSAs, instead, resemble conventional adenomas [21]. TSAs usually locate in the distal colon, and present a cytoplasmic eosinophilia and tubulovillous architectures [21].

Most SSADs present BRAF mutation. TSAs, instead, are more frequently associated with KRAS-mutation and likely give rise to microsatellite stable (MSS) cancer through hypermethylation of DNA repair gene MGMT [22]. Dysplasia is found in SSAs that present hyper-methylation of various genes (CIMP) including p16 and MLH1 resulting in early invasive cancer, more aggressive than conventional adenoma of proximal colon [22].

Several studies have put light on the fact that SSADs are at greater risk of progression to colorectal cancer than TSAs, marking the necessity of an adequate surveillance [21]. Dysplasia is a necessary step for progression to malignancy [21]. High grade dysplasia or intramucosal carcinomas have been found in KRAS-mut TSAs [21, 27]. The combination of serrated pathway features like CpG island methylation and the characteristics of the conventional pathway like chromosomal deletion and p53 mutation have been called "fusion pathway polyps" [21, 26, 28].

1.5.4 Mixed Polyps

The World Health Organization defined mixed polyps lesions which have a combination of hyperplastic, classical adenomatous or TSA or sessile serrated lesion components with different grades of intraepithelial neoplasia [1, 2]. The mixed polyps can contain components of SSA and TSA, SSA and conventional adenomas, TSA and conventional adenoma, and rarely HP and conventional adenoma [1]. The different histopathological type must be indicated in the diagnosis [2].

1.6 Mucosal Polyps

Mucosal polyps are small polyps where the submucosa has elevated the normal tissue. They have no clinical significance [3].

1.7   Juvenile Polyps

Juvenile polyps are solitary, spherical polyps that usually are located in the rectum of children [2, 3]. They show an excess of lamina propria and have cystic dilated glands [2]. In juvenile polyps, neoplasia is rare but they often show hyperplasia [2]. They are also known as retention polyps for the distended, mucus-filled glands, inflammatory cells, and edematous lamina propria [3, 29].

1.8   Peutz-Jeghers's polyps

Peutz–Jeghers polyps are usually present in Peutz–Jeghers syndrome and rarely as single polyps [2]. Polyps have a very organized structure consisting in a central core smooth muscle with conspicuous branching covered by hyperplastic colorectal mucosa [2].

Differently from juvenile polyps, in Peutz–Jeghers polyps the lamina propria is normal and the abnormal muscle tissue confer the characteristic architecture of the lesion [3].

1.9   Inflammatory Polyps

Inflammatory polyps are associated with inflammatory bowel disease, diverticulosis, and mucosal prolapse [2]. Inflammatory polyps are thought to originate after mucosal inflammation with full thickness ulceration and tissue regeneration [30]. Inflammatory polyps might represent island of inflamed edematous mucosa with granulation tissue in the middle of mucosal ulceration [30]. These polyps have no intrinsic neoplastic potential, but they often appear in diseased colons that are at high risk to develop colon cancer [30].

1.10   Malignant Polyps

Malignant polyps are adenomatous growth containing transformed cells that have invaded the submucosa [31]. Such malignant polyps are found in 0.2–9% of endoscopically removed adenomatous polyps [32].

Higher rates of malignancy have been reported in villous adenomas (10–18%) compared with tubulovillous (6–8%) and tubular (2–3%) types [33].

Endoscopically, the presence of depressed ulceration, irregular contour, deformity, a short and immobile stalk, and the inability to elevate sessile polyp upon submucosa bleb formation must put in alert endoscopist [31].

The diagnosis of malignancy is ultimately histological [31]. There are several histological features which have been suggested to associate with higher probability of residual disease or recurrent carcinoma [32, 33]. The diagnosis and the oncological risk are defined by these elements: histological grade, lymphovascular invasion, tumor budding, margin of resection, and microstadiation [33]. There are four different levels of tumor differentiation from G1 (well differentiated) to G4 (undifferentiated). For therapeutic purposes, these levels are further divided into low-grade malignant polyps (G1 and G2) and high-grade malignant polyps (G3 and G4) [34]. Lymphatic invasion by cancer is defined as tumor cells visible within a true endothelial channel in absence of erythrocytes [33]. CD31 or CD34 marker could help in assessing vascular invasion especially if there are fixation artifacts in paraffin sections [33]. Tumor budding describes the presence of isolated single cancer cells or small cluster of cancer cells (less than 5 cells) at the advancing edge of the tumor [33, 34]. Tumors are positive for budding if they present five or more buds per 20 power fields [33]. There is increasing evidence that the presence of tumor budding reflects clinical aggressiveness of colon cancer and it is associated with lymph node metastasis and other adverse outcomes [33, 35]. Ensuring a histologically assessed resection margin free of cancer is very important. Cancer cells present near (less than a 1 mm) the resection margin or within diathermocoagulation line on histological examination increase the risk for an adverse outcome [33, 34]. Finally, microstadiation permits to recognize lesions of different metastatic potential. Histologically, polyps are classified by different factors but probably the most important characteristic is the depth of invasion [35]. There are two schemes to evaluate tumor invasion: Haggitt and Kikuchi scheme. Haggitt classification system for pedunculated and sessile polyps is an important prognostic factor. Pedunculated polyps can be classified as level 0–4.

- Level 0 suggests that cancer cells are restricted to the mucosa and do not enter the muscularis mucosae [35, 36].
- Levels 1 indicates cancer cells invading into the submucosa but limited to the head of the polyps [33, 35, 36].
- Level 2 is present when carcinoma invades the level of the neck (the junction of the head and stalk) [33, 35, 36].
- Level 3 signifies that cancer cells invade any part of the stalk [33, 35, 36].
- Level 4 indicates that cancer cells invade into the submucosa of the bowel wall below the stalk but above the muscularis propria of the polyps [33, 35, 36].

Sessile adenomas with any degree of invasion that give rise to invasive cancer are defined as level 4 [33, 35, 36].

The submucosal invasion of adenocarcinoma in sessile polyps was further classified by Kudo [37] and Kikuchi [38]. They classified submucosal invasion into three levels: Sm1 in case of invasion of the upper third of submucosa; Sm2 invasion into the middle third of the mucosa; Sm3 invasion into the lower third of the mucosa [35]. Kikuchi and colleagues further modified the classification deepening Sm1 classification: SM1a less than a quarter of the width of the tumor invading the submucosa; SM1b between a quarter and a half of the width of the tumor invading the submucosa; SM1c more than a half of the width of the tumor invading the submucosa [33]. This classification is difficult to use if histological samples do not include a significant portion of the submucosa or some of the muscularis propria [35] (Fig. 1.1). On the basis of these criteria it is possible to differentiate malignant polyps at high or low grade of metastasis risk (Table 1.3).

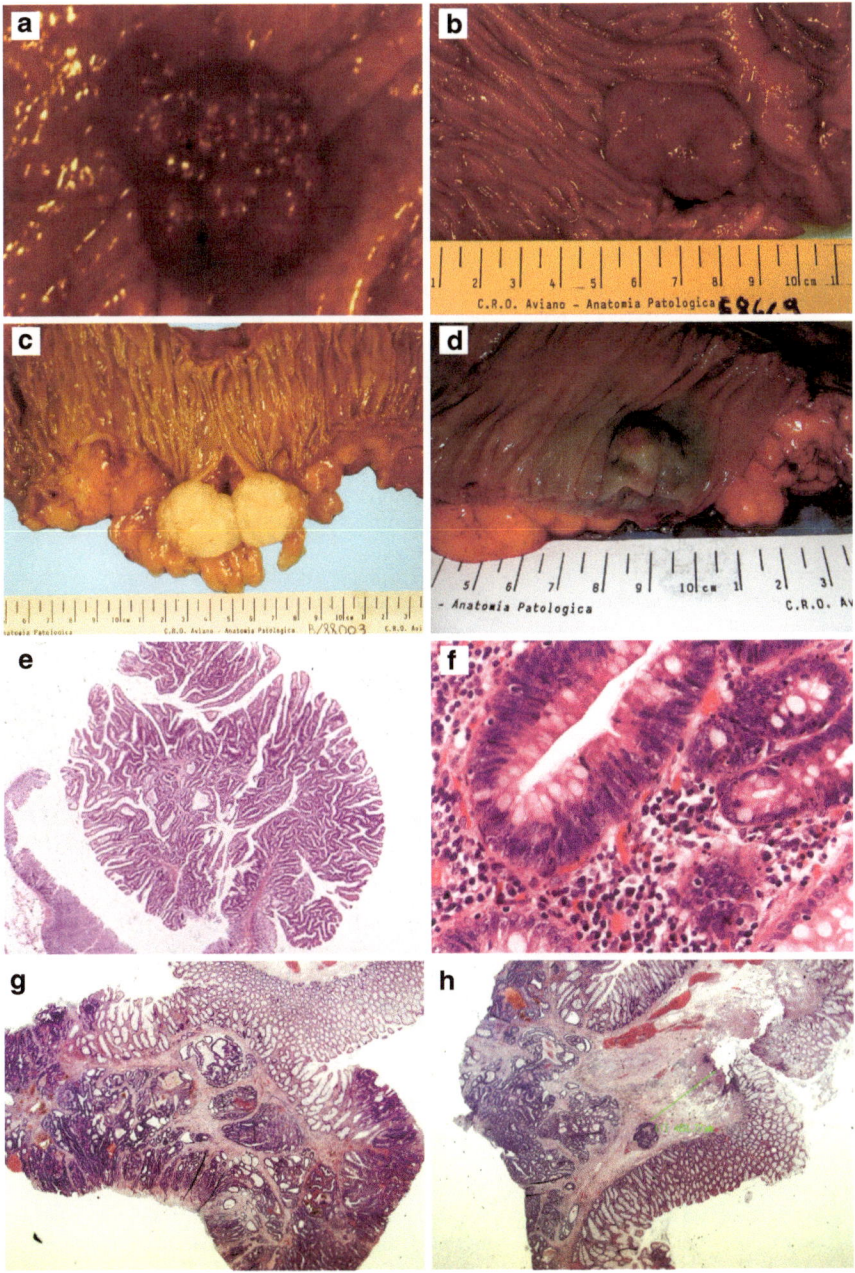

Fig. 1.1 (**a**) Macroscopic appearance of tubular adenoma; (**b**) macroscopic appearance of polypoid sessile adenocarcinoma in tubular adenoma; (**c**) macroscopic appearance of pedunculated lipomatous polypoid lesion with lobulated yellow cut surface; (**d**) macroscopic appearance of residual mucosa after polyp endoscopic removal; (**e**) histological features of tubulovillous pedunculated adenoma; (**f**) low-grade epithelial dysplasia in adenomatous polyp; (**g**) malignant polyps: adenocarcinoma in tubular adenoma. The malignant neoplastic proliferation invades the upper third of submucosa; (**h**) micrometric evaluation of distance of neoplastic cells from the resection margin

Table 1.3 Malignant polyps classification: low-grade or high-grade risk of metastasis	Malignant polyp "low-grade" Grade G1–G2	Malignant polyp "high-grade" Grade G3–G4
	Resection margin >1 mm	Infiltration at <1 mm
	No lymphovascular invasion	Lymphovascular invasion
	Haggitt levels 1–3	Haggitt levels 3–4
	Sm invasion <1 mm	Sm invasion >1 mm
	Size of invasion <4 mm and depth <2 mm	Size of invasion >4 mm and depth >2 mm
	En-bloc resection	Tumor budding
		Piecemeal removal

Modified from "Il polipo cancerizzato" and "Management of malignant colon polyps: current status and controversies" [34, 35]

References

1. Aust DE, Baretton GB, Members of the Working Group GI-pathology of the German Society of Pathology. Serrated polyps of the colon and rectum (hyperplastic polyps, sessile serrated adenomas, traditional serrated adenomas, and mixed polyps)-proposal for diagnostic criteria. Virchows Arch. 2010;457(3):291–7.
2. Segnan N, Patnick J, von Karsa L, editors. European Guidelines for quality assurance in colorectal cancer screening and diagnosis. 1st ed. Luxembourg, Pubblication Office of the European Union; 2010. p. 386.
3. The Paris endoscopic classification of superficial neoplastic lesions: esophagus, stomach, and colon: November 30 to December 1, 2002. Gastrointest Endosc. 2003;58(6 Suppl):S3–43. Review.
4. Strum WB. Colorectal adenomas. N Engl J Med. 2016;374(11):1065–75.
5. Konishi F, Morson BC. Pathology of colorectal adenomas: a colonoscopic survey. J Clin Pathol. 1989;35:830.
6. Bosman F, Yan P. Molecular pathology of colorectal cancer. Pol J Pathol. 2014;65(4):257–66.
7. Fearon ER, Vogelstein B. A genetic model for colorectal carcinogenesis. Cell. 1996;87:159–70.
8. De Sousa E Melo F, Wang X, Jansen M, et al. Poor-prognosis colon cancer is defined by a molecularly distinct subtype and develops from serrated precursor lesions. Nat Med. 2013;19:614–8.
9. Budinska E, Popovici V, Tejpar S, et al. Gene expression patterns unveil a new level of molecular heterogeneity in colorectal cancer. J Pathol. 2013;231:63–76.
10. Arvelo F, Sojo F, Cotte C. Biology of colorectal cancer. Ecancermedicalscience. 2015;9:520.
11. Worthley DL, Leggett BA. Colorectal cancer: molecular features and clinical opportunities. Clin Biochem Rev. 2010;31(2):31–8.
12. Fleming NI, Jorissen RN, Mouradov D, et al. SMAD2, SMAD3 and SMAD4 mutations in colorectal cancer. Crit Rev Oncol Hematol. 2011;79:1–16.
13. Fearon ER, Vogelstein B. A genetic model for colorectal tumorigenesis. Cell. 1990;61(5):759–67.
14. Laurent-Puig P, Agostini J, Maley K. Colorectal oncogenesis bull. Cancer. 2010;97:13.
15. Arrington AK, Heinrich EL, Lee W, Duldulao M, Patel S, Sanchez J, Garcia-Aguilar J, Kim J. Prognostic and predictive roles of KRAS mutation in colorectal cancer. Int J Mol Sci. 2012;13(10):12153–68.
16. Powell SM, Zilz N, Beazer-Barclay Y, et al. APC mutations occur early during colorectal tumorigenesis. Nature. 1992;359:235–7.
17. Nyström-Lahti M, Parsons R, Sistonen P, et al. Mismatch repair genes on chromosomes 2p and 3p account for a major share of hereditary nonpolyposis colorectal cancer families evaluable by linkage. Am J Hum Genet. 1994;55:659–65.

18. Loeb LA. Cancer cells exhibit a mutator phenotype. Adv Cancer Res. 1998;72:25–56.
19. Cunningham JM, Christensen ER, Tester DJ, et al. Hypermethylation of the hMLH1 promoter in colon cancer with microsatellite instability. Cancer Res. 1998;58:3455–60.
20. Beggs AD, et al. Whole-genome methylation analysis of benign and malignant colorectal tumours. J Pathol. 2013;229(5):697–704.
21. Huang CS, Farraye FA, Yang S, O'Brien MJ. The clinical significance of serrated polyps. Am J Gastroenterol. 2011;106(2):229–40.
22. Okamoto K, Kitamura S, Kimura T, Nakagawa T, Sogabe M, Miyamoto H, Muguruma N, Takayama T. Clinicopathological characteristics of serrated polyps as precursors to colorectal cancer: current status and management. J Gastroenterol Hepatol. 2017;32(2):358–67.
23. Spring KJ, Zhao ZZ, Karamatic R, Walsh MD, Whitehall VL, Pike T, Simms LA, Young J, James M, Montgomery GW, Appleyard M, Hewett D, Togashi K, Jass JR, Leggett BA. High prevalence of sessile serrated adenomas with BRAF mutations: a prospective study of patients undergoing colonoscopy. Gastroenterology. 2006;131(5):1400–7.
24. Leggett B, Whitehall V. Role of the serrated pathway in colorectal cancer pathogenesis. Gastroenterology. 2010;138(6):2088–100.
25. Jass JR. Serrated adenoma of the colorectum and the DNA-methylator phenotype. Nat Clin Pract Oncol. 2005;2:398–405.
26. Snover DC. Update on the serrated pathway to colorectal carcinoma. Hum Pathol. 2011;42:1–10.
27. Kim KM, Lee EJ, Kim YH, Chang DK, Odze RD. KRAS mutations in traditional serrated adenomas from Korea herald an aggressive phenotype. Am J Surg Pathol. 2010;34(5):667–75.
28. Jass JR, Baker K, Zlobec I, Higuchi T, Barker M, Buchanan D, Young J. Advanced colorectal polyps with the molecular and morphological features of serrated polyps and adenomas: concept of a 'fusion' pathway to colorectal cancer. Histopathology. 2006;49(2):121–31.
29. Calva D, Howe JR. Hamartomatous polyposis syndromes. Surg Clin North Am. 2008;88(4):779–817.
30. Syal G, Budhraja V. Recurrent obstructive giant inflammatory polyposis of the colon. ACG Case Rep J. 2016;3(4):e89.
31. Hassan C, Zullo A, Winn S, Eramo A, Tomao S, Rossini FP, Morini S. The colorectal malignant polyp: scoping a dilemma. Dig Liver Dis. 2007;39(1):92–100.
32. Netzer P, Forster C, Biral R, Ruchti C, Neuweiler J, Stauffer E, Schönegg R, Maurer C, Hüsler J, Halter F, Schmassmann A. Risk factor assessment of endoscopically removed malignant colorectal polyps. Gut. 1998;43(5):669–74.
33. Williams JG, Pullan RD, Hill J, Horgan PG, Salmo E, Buchanan GN, Rasheed S, McGee SG, Haboubi N, Association of Coloproctology of Great Britain and Ireland. Management of the malignant colorectal polyp: ACPGBI position statement. Colorectal Dis. 2013;15(Suppl 2):1–38.
34. Marini M, Lazzi S. Il polipo cancerizzato. Giorn Ital End Dig. 2014;37:263–8.
35. Aarons CB, Shanmugan S, Bleier JI. Management of malignant colon polyps: current status and controversies. World J Gastroenterol. 2014;20(43):16178–83.
36. Haggitt RC, Glotzbach RE, Soffer EE, Wruble LD. Prognostic factors in colorectal carcinomas arising in adenomas: implications for lesions removed by endoscopic polypectomy. Gastroenterology. 1985;89:328–36.
37. Kudo S. Endoscopic mucosal resection of flat and depressed types of early colorectal cancer. Endoscopy. 1993;25:455–61.
38. Kikuchi R, Takano M, Takagi K, Fujimoto N, Nozaki R, Fujiyoshi T, Uchida Y. Management of early invasive colorectal cancer. Risk of recurrence and clinical guidelines. Dis Colon Rectum. 1995;38:1286–95.

Methods to Improve the Adenoma Detection Rate

2

Vasilios Papadopoulos and Konstantinos Triantafyllou

2.1   Introduction

Colorectal cancer (CRC) is the second most prevalent cause of human cancer-related deaths in Europe [1], and the third in the United States [2]. To date, colonoscopy represents the optimal procedure for CRC screening, since it provides the opportunity of detection and subsequent removal of adenomatous polyps, thus, reducing the incidence and mortality of CRC [3, 4]. However, colonoscopy suffers from several imperfections. Back to back colonoscopy studies have shown that up to 25% of adenomas are missed during colonoscopy, resulting in high interval cancer incidence [5, 6].

In light of these observations, a high-quality examination that will ensure the detection and removal of all precancerous lesions is warranted, and so several quality assessment indicators have been developed, such as the worldwide-accepted adenoma detection rate (ADR), and continuous quality improvement programs have been implemented [7]. ADR is defined as the proportion of average-risk patients undergoing first-time screening colonoscopy in which at least one adenoma is found. It has been demonstrated that ADR correlates directly with interval cancer (CRC after negative colonoscopy), as an ADR that exceeds 25% is significantly associated with a reduction in interval CRC [8]. Moreover, ADR has been inversely associated with the risk of advanced-stage interval cancer and fatal interval cancer [9]. Current ASGE guidelines propose that in patients undergoing screening colonoscopy, an ADR of $\geq 30\%$ in men and of $\geq 20\%$ in women should be achieved, at least [10].

V. Papadopoulos • K. Triantafyllou (✉)
Hepatogastroenterology Unit, Second Department of Internal Medicine—Propaedeutic, Research Institute and Diabetes Center, Medical School, National and Kapodistrian University, Attikon University General Hospital, 1 Rimini Street, 124 62 Athens, Greece
e-mail: ktriant@med.uoa.gr

© Springer International Publishing AG 2018
A. Facciorusso, N. Muscatiello (eds.), *Colon Polypectomy*,
https://doi.org/10.1007/978-3-319-59457-6_2

In this chapter, we will highlight various procedural and technical-dependent factors that contribute to ADR improvement.

2.2 Procedure-Related Factors

The evidences listed below are summarized in Table 2.1.

Table 2.1 Studies evaluating the impact of pre- and intra-procedural issues on adenoma detection rate

Author (year) [ref]	Method	Study design	N	ADR	Limitations
Oh (2015) [11]	Overall bowel preparation quality	Single-center retrospective study	6097	OR: 0.55 (95%CI 0.41–0.75) for poor/fair preparation	Study design
Gurudu (2012) [15]	Same-day vs. split-dose preparation	Single-center retrospective study	3560 vs. 1615	26.7 vs. 31.8%	Study design Different endoscopists per period
Clark (2014) [16]	Overall bowel preparation quality	Meta-analysis	31,047 vs. 4058	OR: 1.30 (95%CI 1.19–1.42) favoring adequate vs. inadequate preparation	Different bowel preparation quality scales used
Adler (2012) [17]	Overall bowel preparation quality	Multicenter prospective cohort study from private practice	12,134	OR: 0.64 (95%CI 0.47–0.87) for poor preparation and OR: 0.22 (95%CI 0.05–0.92) for insufficient preparation	Relatively small number of participating colonoscopists
Tholey (2015) [18]	Overall bowel preparation quality	Single-center retrospective cross-sectional study	5113	OR: 0.97 (95%CI 0.85–1.11) for excellent preparation	Study design
Clark (2016) [19]	Overall bowel preparation quality	Single-center prospective study	749	OR: 0.37 (95%CI 0.15–0.87) favoring high-quality preparation in detecting sessile adenomas	Male population exclusively

Table 2.1 (continued)

Author (year) [ref]	Method	Study design	N	ADR	Limitations
Calderwood (2015) [20]	Overall bowel preparation quality	Two-center retrospective cross-sectional study	Center A: 3713	OR: 1.3 (95%CI 1.1–1.6) for good preparation	Retrospective study
Barcley (2006) [21]	Withdrawal time	Prospective cohort study	2053	28.3 vs. 11.8% (mean WT: ≥6 min vs. <6 min)	Study design
Jover (2013) [22]	Withdrawal time	Multicenter prospective observational study	4539	OR: 1.51 (95%CI 1.17–1.96) for mean WT >8 min	Study design
Butterly (2014) [23]	Withdrawal time	Retrospective study	7996	OR: 1.50 (95%CI 1.21–1.85) for WT = 9 min	Study design. Withdrawal time recorded by performer
Lee (2013) [24]	Withdrawal time	Retrospective study	31,088	42.5 vs. 47.1% (mean WT < 7 vs. ≥11 min)	Study design. Only FOB-positive participants
Vavricka (2016) [25]	Withdrawal time	Single-center prospective study	355 vs. 203	21.4 vs. 36% for monitored-unaware vs. monitored-aware performers	Short-term study
Kushnir (2015) [29]	Second RC inspection (second pass vs. retroflexion)	Two-center prospective randomized parallel controlled study	400 vs. 455	46 vs. 47%, both methods leaded to incremental ADR	Academicals medical centers
Lee (2016) [30]	Retroflexion following two forward-viewing RC examination	Single-center prospective cohort study	1020	25.5% after two FV examinations vs. 27.5% third pass with RV	Non-randomized
Triantafyllou (2016) [31]	Retroflexion following forward-viewing RC examination	Single-center prospective cohort study	674	6.6% ADR increase	Non-randomized
Ramirez (2011) [34]	Water-aided colonoscopy	Single-center randomized prospective study	177 vs. 191	57.1% WAC vs. 46.1% AI	Single unblinded endoscopist

(continued)

Table 2.1 (continued)

Author (year) [ref]	Method	Study design	N	ADR	Limitations
Hsieh (2014) [36]	Water-aided colonoscopy	Single-center prospective randomized study	90 vs. 90 vs. 90	Overall ADR: 45.6% WI vs. 56.7% WE vs. 43.3% AIC RC ADR: 14.4% WI vs. 26.7% WE vs. 11.1% AIC	Single unblinded endoscopist
Cadoni (2014) [37]	Water-aided colonoscopy	Two-center prospective randomized study	338 vs. 334	25.8% WAC vs. 19.1% AI	Low ADR
Hsieh (2016) [38]	Water-aided colonoscopy	Two-center prospective randomized study	217 vs. 217 vs. 217	Overall ADR: 40.6% WI vs. 49.8% WE vs. 37.8 AI RC ADR: 17.5% WI vs. 21.7% WE vs. 15.3% AI	Long WE insertion time
Xu (2016) [39]	Nurse participation	RCTs meta-analysis	1672 (3 studies)	45.7% nurse participating vs. 39.3% colonoscopist alone	Small number of RCTs included
Chalifoux (2014) [40]	Trainee participation	Single-center retrospective study	2250 (SD: 1080 HD: 1170)	SD group: 47% without trainee vs. 50% with trainee HD group: 51% without trainee vs. 63% with trainee	Single-center study, lack of WT documentation
Buchner (2011) [41]	Trainee participation	Single-center retrospective study	2430	Overall ADR: 26% without trainee vs. 30% with trainee Diminutive ADR: 17% without trainee vs. 25% with trainee	Lack of data regarding bowel preparation
Gianotti (2016) [42]	Fellow participation	Single-center retrospective study	919 vs. 1806	25% without fellow vs. 36% with fellow with experience of >140 colonoscopies	Low ADR of the attending only colonoscopy

ADR adenoma detection rate, *WT* withdrawal time, *FOB* fecal occult blood, *RC* right colon, *FV* forward-view, *RV* retroflexion-view, *WAC* water-aided colonoscopy, *AI* air insufflation, *WE* water exchange, *WI* water immersion, *AI* air insufflation, *SD* standard-definition, *HD* high-definition

2.2.1 Bowel Preparation

While bowel preparation prior to colonoscopy is described by many patients as the most difficult and unpleasant part of the procedure, inadequate bowel preparation has been linked to low ADR [11]. Bowel reparation is considered adequate when the endoscopist is allowed to detect lesions greater than 5 mm in size in every colon segment [12]. Recent guidelines by the European Society of Gastrointestinal Endoscopy [13] and the American Society for Gastrointestinal Endoscopy [14], regarding bowel preparation before colonoscopy, provide useful guidance on this matter. First, split-dose preparation is strongly recommended, as it has been associated with ADR improvement [15]. The second dose of purgatives should be administrated between 3 and 8 h prior the procedure according to ASGE and 4 h according to ESGE. Same-day preparation should be encouraged only for colonoscopies scheduled in the afternoon. Second, a low-residue diet is preferable the day before the examination. Third, oral and written instructions regarding preparation should be provided to each patient, emphasizing on the necessity of adequate bowel preparation. Finally, while 4 L polyethylene glycol (PEG) is considered superior against all other bowel preparation compounds, the optimal choice of formulation should be individualized.

It seems logical that improving the bowel cleansing will yield higher ADRs. There is compelling evidence supporting this association [16, 17]. However, it is uncertain if there is any significant improvement in ADR as the degree of bowel cleanliness improves from good to excellent. A few studies have found that high-quality bowel preparation is associated with a superior detection of advanced adenomas and sessile serrated polyps [18, 19]. On the contrary, results from a retrospective study reported only marginal decrease in ADR at the highest levels of bowel cleansing [20]. Authors suggested that an excellent preparation may provide a false sense of overconfidence to endoscopists and led to less meticulous inspection of the colonic mucosa.

2.2.2 Withdrawal Time

Various studies have detected that longer time of withdrawal is associated with higher ADR [21, 22]. Current guidelines recommend that 6 min is the minimum length of time that allows adequate observation of the colonic mucosa during the instrument withdrawal [10], while a longer withdrawal time of 9 min further increases ADR [23]. On the other hand, a withdrawal time prolonged beyond 10 min is associated with a minimal increase in ADR [24].

It is important to state that endoscopists who take longer to withdraw the endoscope do not necessarily have a high-quality colonoscopic withdrawal technique. The withdrawal time should be spent carefully to improve the visualization of the colonic mucosa. Examination of the proximal sides of flexures and folds, thorough washing of the mucosa and suction of debris, alert visualization, and adequate distention of colon are of paramount importance. Additionally, systematic monitoring of the withdrawal time may improve ADR as it has been shown that ADR increases significantly when endoscopists are aware of being supervised during the examination [25].

2.2.3 Second Right Colon Inspection

Incontrovertible evidence point out that colonoscopy is less effective in preventing right-sided colon cancer [26]. Several reasons could be held accountable. First, right-sided polyps are mostly serrated lesions and adenomas with flat morphology and thus more difficult to detect. In addition, polyps are frequently located on the proximal aspects of haustral folds and the area around the hepatic flexure. These sites often remain hidden from standard forward-viewing colonoscopes. Therefore, it is essential to improve the performance of colonoscopy in the proximal colon. A simple and inexpensive method of improving the diagnostic yield of the procedure is the second inspection of the right colon, either by implementation of the retroflexion maneuver [27] or by a second forward-view examination [28]. Results from a prospective study reported that using either one of the aforementioned techniques has incremental benefit on ADR [29], while another study demonstrated that retroflexion in the proximal colon achieves higher ADR, even after two consecutive forward-view examinations [30]. On the contrary, a prospective cohort study that included 674 procedures did not demonstrate any significant benefit regarding right colon adenoma detection by the implementation of the retroflexion maneuver [31].

2.2.4 Water-Aided Colonoscopy

Water infusion methods including the water immersion (WI) and the water exchange (WE) have been proposed to decrease discomfort and minimize sedation use during colonoscopy [32]. Both methods infuse water to distend colon during insertion. In WI, infused water is adjunct to air insufflation, and it is removed predominantly during withdrawal of the scope. In WE, added water is immediately removed during insertion and combined with exclusion of air insufflation and suction of residual air.

Apart from that, water-aided colonoscopy has demonstrated further advantages. Several studies including systematic reviews have compared the water infusion methods with standard air insufflation, evaluating among others screening efficacy [33–35]. Water-aided colonoscopy was associated with a higher ADR, particularly in the right colon [34, 36, 37]. These results can be explained by the observation that intermittent water infusion may clean the mucosa better and thus allow the endoscopist to devote a greater proportion of the withdrawal time to inspection. Furthermore, polyps are prone to better visualization in a water-filled colon because of being less flattened, combined with the magnifying effect of water.

Finally, a head-to-head prospective randomized study with ADR as primary outcome found that WE compared with air insufflation significantly increased ADR (49.8 vs. 37.8%, $p = 0.016$), while there was no difference between WE and WI [38]. Authors suggested that the role of WE method in CRC prevention should be further assessed. However, ADR improvement can be attributed to the longer WE insertion time, thus longer inspection time.

2.2.5   Second Investigator

The presence of an endoscopy nurse or trainee during colonoscopy can improve ADR. Several explanations have been proposed for this association. Even when a lesion is within the field of view, the endoscopist may miss it. This may be due to fail to detect change in the visual field as long as the change occurs during an eye movement or interruptions of visual scanning. Addition of a second observer may improve the attentiveness of the endoscopist, due to a form of competition between the two observers.

A meta-analysis of three randomized controlled trials evaluating nurse participation in colonoscopy observation showed a significant higher ADR in the nurse presence group than endoscopist alone (45.7 vs. 39.3%) [39]. Results in trainees' participation studies are similar. In a retrospective study, trainee participation during screening colonoscopies, performed with standard or high-definition colonoscopes significantly improved ADR but only when colonoscopies were performed with high-definition scopes [40]. In a similar manner, results from a retrospective study showed that trainee participation improves only detection of diminutive adenomas (<5 mm) [41]. Of note, ADR of fellows who had performed >140 colonoscopies under attending supervision has been found to exceed that of the attenders (36 vs. 25%, $p < 0.0001$) [42]. In conclusion, it is difficult to evade the conclusion that routine observation of colonoscopy withdrawal by a second investigator can improve ADR.

2.3   Technological-Related Factors

2.3.1   Accessory Devices

During the last decade, several endoscopic innovations aiming to enhance visualization behind colonic folds and curves have been developed. We will describe the main accessory devices that either flatten colonic folds or enable a direct view behind them. The current evidence is summarized in Table 2.2.

2.3.1.1 Cap-Assisted Colonoscopy
A transparent plastic cap is attached to the distal tip of the colonoscope in cap-assisted colonoscopy (CAC), depressing the haustral folds and improving mucosal exposure. Moreover, the cap retains the tip of the scope a sufficient distance away from the mucosa allowing the endoscopist to preserve a continuous visual area around the colonic bends. The diameter of the cap depends on the size of the scope, while cap protrusion varies from 2 to 10 mm with 4-mm-long cap used in most studies. In recent years, cap utilization has become popular among endoscopists, especially trainees, as this technique decreases patient discomfort and cecal intubation time [43], while it increases cecal intubation rate [44].

However, there are conflicting data regarding the impact of cap utilization in ADR. There is some evidence that cap-fitted colonoscopy is more effective than standard colonoscopy (SC) in terms of ADR (69 vs. 56%, $p = 0.009$) [45], especially

Table 2.2 Studies evaluating the impact of add-on devices and new endoscopes on adenoma detection rate

Author (year) [ref]	Technology	Study design	N	ADR (%)	AMR (%)	Limitations
Rastogi (2012) [45]	CAC vs. SC	Single-center prospective randomized parallel design	210 vs. 210	69 vs. 56	NA	Investigator bias in favor of CAC
Kim (2015) [46]	CAC vs. SC	Single-center retrospective parallel design	515 vs. 508	35.7 vs. 28.3	NA	Longer withdrawal time in CAC group
Pohl (2015) [47]	CAC vs. SC	Two-center randomized parallel design	561 vs. 552	42 vs. 40	NA	Limited prior experience with cap
Lee (2009) [48]	CAC vs. SC	Two-center prospective randomized parallel design	499 vs. 501	30.5 vs. 37.5	NA	Inadequate sample
Ng (2012) [49]	CAC vs. SC	Meta-analysis	726 vs. 707 (six studies)	46.8 vs. 45.3	NA	Absence of polyp histology in most studies
Lenze (2014) [51]	Endocuff	Single-center retrospective	50	34	NA	No comparator
Biecker (2015) [52]	Endocuff vs. SC	Two-center prospective randomized parallel design	245 vs. 253	36 vs. 28	NA	Small sample. Withdrawal times not measured
Floer (2014) [53]	Endocuff vs. SC	Multicenter prospective randomized parallel design	249 vs. 242	35.4 vs. 20.7	NA	Small sample
Van Doorn (2015) [54]	Endocuff vs. SC	Two-center prospective randomized parallel design	504 vs. 529	54 vs. 53	NA	Inadequate sample. Study restricted on experts
Chin (2016) [55]	Endocuff vs. SC	Meta-analysis	4387 (eight studies)	50.4 vs. 43.3	NA	Tandem studies not included
Triantafyllou (2016) [56]	Endocuff vs. SC	Multicenter prospective randomized tandem study	100 vs. 100	NA	14.7 vs. 37.6	ADR not measured
Dik (2015) [58]	EndoRings vs. SC	Multicenter prospective randomized tandem study	57 vs. 59	49.1 vs. 28.8[a]	10.4 vs. 48.3	Inadequate sample to measure ADR
Granlek (2014) [59]	G-EYE	Single-center prospective cohort	47	44.7	NA	No comparator

Table 2.2 (continued)

Author (year) [ref]	Technology	Study design	N	ADR (%)	AMR (%)	Limitations
Halpern (2014) [60]	G-EYE vs. SC	Multicenter prospective randomized parallel design	54 vs. 52	40.4 vs. 25.9	7.5 vs. 44.7	Inadequate sample to measure ADR
Rubin (2015) [61]	TEP/SC[b]	Single-center prospective feasibility	33	44	NA	No comparator
Granlek (2014) [63]	FUSE vs. SC	Multicenter prospective randomized tandem study	101 vs. 96	34 vs. 28[a]	7 vs. 41	Inadequate sample to measure ADR
Papanikolaou (2017) [64]	FUSE vs. SC/R	Two-center prospective randomized tandem study	107 vs. 108	NA	10.9 vs. 33.7	ADR not measured. Protocol violation cases replaced with new ones
Hassan (2016) [65]	FUSE vs. SC	Multicenter prospective randomized parallel design	328 vs. 330	43.6 vs. 45.5	NA	Inadequate sample size for primary endpoint. Only FIT-positive cases. Only expert endoscopists

NA non-applicable, *ADR* adenoma detection rate, *AMR* adenoma miss rate, *SC* standard colonoscopy, *SC/R* standard colonoscopy plus examination of the right colon with scope retroflexion, *TEP* third-eye panoramic view, *CAC* cap-assisted colonoscopy, *FUSE* full-spectrum endoscopy system
[a]Refers to the first of the tandem examinations
[b]Concomitant use of TEP and SC

in the right colon (29 vs. 16.9%, $p < 0.001$) [46]. On the other hand, a large randomized study comparing CAC to standard colonoscopy failed to find any difference in ADR between the two procedures (42 vs. 40%, $p = 0.452$) [47]. Furthermore, a study reported that the ADR in CAC group was significantly lower than that in the standard group (30.5 vs 37.5%, $p = 0.02$), thus questioning its efficacy [48].

To overcome these conflicting results, a meta-analysis of 16 randomized clinical trials including 8991 patients aiming to evaluate the efficacy of CAC compared to that of standard colonoscopy in polyp detection and cecal intubation time was conducted [49]. Among the 16 studies, only six reported on ADR as an outcome. Authors concluded that there was no significant difference in terms of ADR between CAC and SC (46.8 vs. 45.3%) although a higher proportion of patients with polyp(s) were detected in the CAC group. In subgroup analysis, a short cap (≤ 4 mm) significantly increased polyp detection, whereas a long cap (≥ 7 mm) significantly reduced cecal intubation time, as well as, total colonoscopy time.

In conclusion, although cap utilization may be beneficial for young endoscopists, cap-assisted colonoscopy has a marginal benefit only in polyp detection rate.

2.3.1.2 Endocuff

In 2011, a new endoscopic device aiming to improve ADR and control of the tip of the colonoscope was introduced. The Endocuff (EC; Arc Medical Design Ltd., Leeds, England) is a 2-cm-long cap designed to be attached to the tip of colonoscope. It features two circular rows of soft and flexible arms that remain flattened during insertion and protrude out on withdrawal, straightening the mucosal folds. More thoroughly, during forward motion, the elastic slim projections of the cuff are hinged at their bases to not interfere with colonic mucosa. However, ileal intubation may be more difficult. During withdrawal, the wings project out due to contact with the colonic mucosa, stabilizing the position of the endoscope in the center of the lumen and spreading out the colonic folds. Therefore, the proximal side of the folds is exposed, and previously hidden polyps may now be detected (Fig. 2.1).

EC was initially used as a stabilizing tool for complex polyp resection in the sigmoid colon [50]. In 2014, the first study evaluating EC-assisted colonoscopy was published [51]. The ADR was 34% and reached 41% in the subgroup of screening colonoscopy, while 42% of the adenomas were located in the right colon. Since then, various studies have been conducted comparing EC-assisted versus standard colonoscopy. Two of them associated the use of EC with a higher ADR [52, 53], while no difference between the two groups regarding the ADR was reported in one

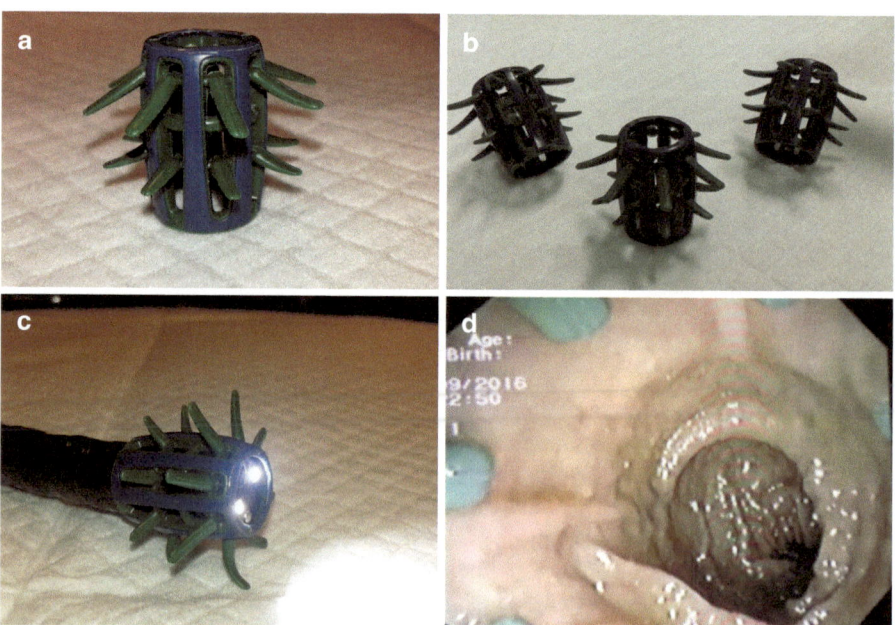

Fig. 2.1 Endocuff (Arc Medical Design Ltd., Leeds, UK) (**a**, **b**); mounted on the colonoscope (**c**); during scope withdrawal the device flattens the colonic folds and its projections may become visible (**d**)

large randomized controlled trial [54]. Finally, a meta-analysis including eight studies which reported ADR as an outcome and 4387 patients has shown superiority of EC-assisted colonoscopy in relation to ADR [55]. A recently presented multicenter tandem study showed for the first time that EC use was related with lower rates of missed adenomas compared to SC (14.7 vs. 37.6%, $p = 0.0004$) [56].

The most commonly reported complication of the EC use is minor mucosal lacerations without any clinical impact. The new version of EC, Endocuff Vision, has one single row of more rounded and longer projections, thus minimizing the mucosal injury and delivering a better tip control. A prospective, multicenter, randomized controlled trial is currently comparing Endocuff Vision-assisted versus standard colonoscopy in terms of ADR [57].

2.3.1.3 EndoRings

The EndoRings device (EndoAid Ltd., Caesarea, Israel) is another easy-to-use endoscopic add-on attachment with design and use similar to EC, except that it consists of two circular rows of flexible rings. It is mounted on the tip of a colonoscope and, during withdrawal, mechanically stretches the colonic folds and provides centering and control of the endoscope (Fig. 2.2). A multicenter, randomized, tandem colonoscopy study demonstrated that EndoRings-assisted colonoscopy has significantly lower polyp and adenoma miss rate than standard colonoscopy [58]. Also, ADR of the first-pass colonoscopy was higher with EndoRings than without it (49.1 vs. 28.8%, $p = 0.025$).

2.3.1.4 Balloon-Assisted Colonoscopy

A novel balloon-colonoscope system (NaviAid G-EYE; Smart Medical Systems, Ra'anana, Israel) has been recently introduced. The G-EYE system consists of a standard colonoscope of any brand and model and a reusable and inflatable balloon that is permanently integrated 1–2 cm behind its distal end. The balloon is inflated through a dedicated inflation system (NaviAid SPARK^{2}C) that enables, beyond anchoring pressure, three additional intermediate pressure levels and can reach a maximal diameter of 60 mm, when fully inflated. Balloon inflation and deflation is

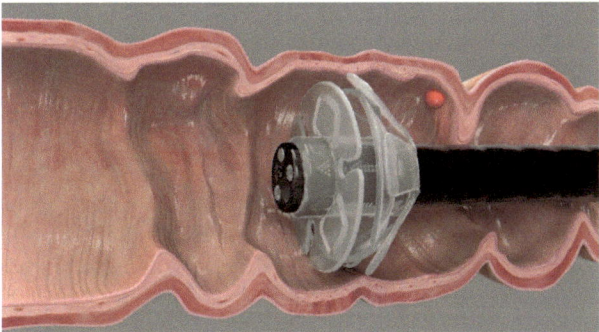

Fig. 2.2 EndoRings (EndoAid Ltd., Caesarea, Israel) mounted on the scope flattens the colonic folds during withdrawal, thus exposing more mucosal area to be examined. Image provided courtesy of EndoAid Ltd., Caesarea, Israel

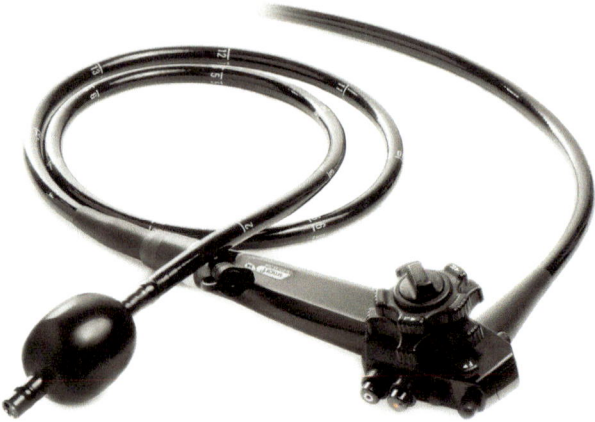

Fig. 2.3 The NaviAid G-EYE (Smart Medical Systems, Ra'anana, Israel). Image provided courtesy of the company

controlled by a foot pedal. When deflated, the diameter of the scope is about 0.1 mm larger than the conventional colonoscope (Fig. 2.3).

During colonoscopy, the scope advances with the balloon deflated. When cecum is reached and examined, the balloon is partially inflated and the balloon colonoscope is withdrawn by the endoscopist like a standard procedure. Withdrawal of the partially inflated balloon flattens the haustral folds, keeps the scope at the center of the lumen, and inhibits bowel slippage during withdrawal. This fold-flattening effect facilitates visualization of the colonic mucosa behind the folds, to increase polyp detection. Moreover, anchoring pressure is enabled when longer stabilization of the colonoscope is needed (e.g., during therapeutic interventions).

A prospective, pilot study tested the safety and feasibility of the G-EYE balloon colonoscope in 50 patients [59]. Authors reported that balloon-assisted colonoscopy had an ADR of 44.7%, and the results of this study were very promising. Consequently, a multicenter, randomized controlled trial with tandem design demonstrated that balloon-assisted colonoscopy was superior to standard colonoscopy regarding adenoma detection (40.4 vs. 25.9%), especially in the ascending colon (40.5 vs. 23.8%) [60]. Authors concluded that this fold-flattening device, due to its increased diagnostic yield, has the potential to reduce interval CRC and, therefore, to fit in the screening programs of endoscopic units.

2.3.1.5 Third-Eye Panoramic

The Third-Eye Panoramic device (TEP; Avantis Medical System, Sunnyvale, USA) is a novel resposable device that enables direct visualization behind colonic folds and flexures. TEP consists of a plastic cap with two video cameras, illuminated by LEDs and directed sideways from its right and left sides, and a flexible plastic catheter containing a video transmission wire. The cap is attached to the tip of any standard colonoscope and holds in place the catheter, which runs alongside the shaft of the endoscope. The proximal end of the catheter plugs into the video processor unit of the colonoscope, and the two lateral images of the TEP are displayed on each side of the scope's forward image, creating a panoramic video image of more than 300°. This wide-angle view allows inspection of the colonic mucosa behind folds and flexures.

A feasibility study [61] reported on the safe and effective use of TEP in 33 patients. TER enabled the visualization of polyps and diverticula which were not initially seen with the scope's forward view. The overall ADR was 44%, but further studies comparing the TEP-assisted to standard colonoscopy, as well as other devices designed to improve ADR, are required.

2.3.2   Wide-Angle Viewing Colonoscopes

Currently, one wide-angle view, the FUSE (EndoChoice, Alpharetta, GA, USA) platform is marketed, while another prototype is close to reach the endoscopy market. The evidence on the performance of these instruments is also summarized in Table 2.2.

2.3.2.1 Full-Spectrum Endoscopy System
Full-Spectrum Endoscopy (FUSE; EndoChoice, Alpharetta, GA, USA) platform consists of a video colonoscope and a main control unit. This novel endoscope has a high-resolution 330° field of view with maintenance of all standard colonoscope capabilities. The full-spectrum view is achieved by using three imagers and light-emitting diode groups positioned at the front and both sides of the forward tip of the scope. Obtained images are displayed on three side-by-side contiguous monitors, thereby creating the 330° field of view and improving visualization of the mucosa behind colonic folds (Fig. 2.4).

Field of View Comparison

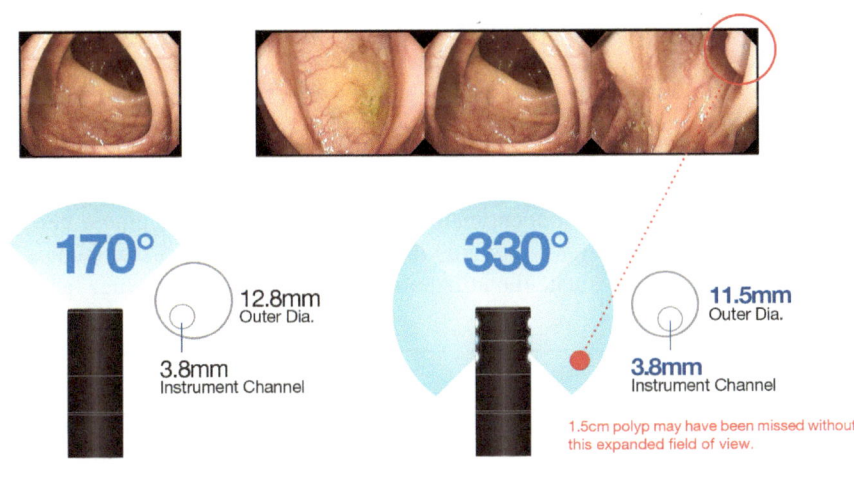

170°
12.8mm Outer Dia.
3.8mm Instrument Channel

330°
11.5mm Outer Dia.
3.8mm Instrument Channel
1.5cm polyp may have been missed without this expanded field of view.

Traditional Colonoscope
Limited 170° Field of View

Fuse® Slim Colonoscope
Panoramic 330° Field of View

Fig. 2.4 Field view comparison between the standard colonoscope and the full-spectrum endoscopy (EndoChoice, Alpharetta, GA, USA). The panoramic 330° of view gives the opportunity to identify lesions with the lateral lenses during withdrawal. Image provided courtesy of the company

Following a successful feasibility study in human subjects [62], an international, multicenter, randomized, tandem study compared the adenoma miss rates of FUSE colonoscopy with those of standard colonoscopy [63]. Per-lesion analysis in 185 patients showed that adenoma miss rate with FUSE colonoscopy was significantly lower than that with standard procedure (7 vs. 41%, $p < 0.001$). Moreover, FUSE detected significantly more adenomas than SC (69% additional adenomas), and most adenomas missed by SC and subsequently detected by FUSE were located in the right colon. In terms of ADR, there was no statistically difference between the two groups due to the small sample size. A recently published study, with similar design to the aforementioned trial, reported a considerably lower overall (10.9 vs. 33.7%, $p < 0.001$) and proximal adenoma miss rate (13.9 vs. 42.2%, $p = 0.006$) with FUSE [64]. It should be mentioned that standard colonoscopy was performed with the addition of right colon reexamination with scope retroflexion.

On the other hand, a large parallel design randomized study enrolling 658 patients undergoing colonoscopy with positive fecal immunochemical test (FIT) demonstrated that FUSE colonoscopy does not increase ADR [65]. More detailed, FIT-positive patients were randomized to undergo either FUSE colonoscopy or SC. No difference in ADR and advanced ADR was detected between the two groups (FUSE 43.6% and 19.5% vs. SC 45.5% and 23.9%, respectively). The inconsistency between the results of this study and the aforementioned tandem studies could be explained by the study design. Parallel group design may be preferable for clinical practice as it compares ADR, but it requires a much larger sample size to achieve adequate statistical power than that of the aforementioned trial [66].

2.3.2.2 Extra-Wide-Angle-View Colonoscope

Extra-wide-angle view colonoscope (Olympus, Tokyo, Japan) is a novel colonoscope with a 13.9-mm tip diameter and a 144–232°-angle backward-lateral view lens in addition to a standard 140°-angle forward-view lens, accompanied by a 180-series processor. The lateral-backward viewing lens is projected in a convex way from the tip of the scope. Images from both lenses are simultaneously presented as a single image on a video monitor. Thus, an extensive surface of colonic mucosa is inspected allowing a more meticulous colon examination.

In a single-arm feasibility study assessing the efficacy and safety of this prototype colonoscope [67], all adenomatous lesions found in the sigmoid colon were first detected by the lateral-backward viewing lens. However, further studies appropriately designed to evaluate the utilization of this novel scope are needed.

2.4   Summary

Colonoscopy is the gold standard for colorectal cancer screening, although a substantial proportion of adenomas are missed during the procedure. ADR is the primary quality indicator to measure effective colonoscopy, and there is an inverse association between interval CRC and ADR. In addition to inborn incommensurable endoscopy skill, various methods have been featured to optimize ADR. Adequate bowel preparation, sufficient withdrawal time exceeding the 6 min, and second visualization of the right colon are among others easy-to-follow procedural factors that have demonstrated ADR improvement. During the last years, several endoscopic technologies have been developed to optimize visualization of the colonic mucosa. Although most of them have demonstrated impressive results regarding polyp detection, their impact in clinical practice is still questionable. Beyond additional costs and training requirements, all these modalities have not proved a significant impact on CRC prevention yet, since the advantage of detecting additional lesions is restricted to small, non-advanced adenomas, so far.

Conflict of Interest Statement The authors declare no conflict of interest related to this publication.

References

1. Ferlay J, Steliarova-Foucher E, Lortet-Tieulent J, Rosso S, Coebergh JW, Comber H, Forman D, Bray F. Cancer incidence and mortality patterns in Europe: estimates for 40 countries in 2012. Eur J Cancer. 2013;49(6):1374–403. https://doi.org/10.1016/j.ejca.2012.12.027.
2. Siegel R, Ma J, Zou Z, Jemal A. Cancer statistics, 2014. CA Cancer J Clin. 2014;64(1):9–29. https://doi.org/10.3322/caac.21208.
3. Winawer SJ, Zauber AG, Ho MN, O'Brien MJ, Gottlieb LS, Sternberg SS, Waye JD, Schapiro M, Bond JH, Panish JF, et al. Prevention of colorectal cancer by colonoscopic polypectomy. The National Polyp Study Workgroup. N Engl J Med. 1993;329(27):1977–81. https://doi.org/10.1056/NEJM199312303292701.
4. Zauber AG, Winawer SJ, O'Brien MJ, Lansdorp-Vogelaar I, van Ballegooijen M, Hankey BF, Shi W, Bond JH, Schapiro M, Panish JF, Stewart ET, Waye JD. Colonoscopic polypectomy and long-term prevention of colorectal-cancer deaths. N Engl J Med. 2012;366(8):687–96. https://doi.org/10.1056/NEJMoa1100370.
5. van Rijn JC, Reitsma JB, Stoker J, Bossuyt PM, van Deventer SJ, Dekker E. Polyp miss rate determined by tandem colonoscopy: a systematic review. Am J Gastroenterol. 2006;101(2):343–50. https://doi.org/10.1111/j.1572-0241.2006.00390.x.
6. Heresbach D, Barrioz T, Lapalus MG, Coumaros D, Bauret P, Potier P, Sautereau D, Boustiere C, Grimaud JC, Barthelemy C, See J, Serraj I, D'Halluin PN, Branger B, Ponchon T. Miss rate for colorectal neoplastic polyps: a prospective multicenter study of back-to-back video colonoscopies. Endoscopy. 2008;40(4):284–90. https://doi.org/10.1055/s-2007-995618.
7. Triantafyllou K, Sioulas AD, Kalli T, Misailidis N, Polymeros D, Papanikolaou IS, Karamanolis G, Ladas SD. Optimized sedation improves colonoscopy quality long-term. Gastroenterol Res Pract. 2015;2015:195093. https://doi.org/10.1155/2015/195093.
8. Kaminski MF, Regula J, Kraszewska E, Polkowski M, Wojciechowska U, Didkowska J, Zwierko M, Rupinski M, Nowacki MP, Butruk E. Quality indicators for colonoscopy and the risk of interval cancer. N Engl J Med. 2010;362(19):1795–803. https://doi.org/10.1056/NEJMoa0907667.
9. Corley DA, Jensen CD, Marks AR, Zhao WK, Lee JK, Doubeni CA, Zauber AG, de Boer J, Fireman BH, Schottinger JE, Quinn VP, Ghai NR, Levin TR, Quesenberry CP. Adenoma detection rate and risk of colorectal cancer and death. N Engl J Med. 2014;370(14):1298–306. https://doi.org/10.1056/NEJMoa1309086.
10. Rex DK, Schoenfeld PS, Cohen J, Pike IM, Adler DG, Fennerty MB, Lieb JG 2nd, Park WG, Rizk MK, Sawhney MS, Shaheen NJ, Wani S, Weinberg DS. Quality indicators for colonoscopy. Gastrointest Endosc. 2015;81(1):31–53. https://doi.org/10.1016/j.gie.2014.07.058.

11. Oh CH, Lee CK, Kim JW, Shim JJ, Jang JY. Suboptimal bowel preparation significantly impairs Colonoscopic detection of non-polypoid colorectal neoplasms. Dig Dis Sci. 2015;60(8):2294–303. https://doi.org/10.1007/s10620-015-3628-6.
12. Johnson DA, Barkun AN, Cohen LB, Dominitz JA, Kaltenbach T, Martel M, Robertson DJ, Boland CR, Giardello FM, Lieberman DA, Levin TR, Rex DK, Cancer USM-STFoC. Optimizing adequacy of bowel cleansing for colonoscopy: recommendations from the US multi-society task force on colorectal cancer. Gastroenterology. 2014;147(4):903–24. https://doi.org/10.1053/j.gastro.2014.07.002.
13. Hassan C, Bretthauer M, Kaminski MF, Polkowski M, Rembacken B, Saunders B, Benamouzig R, Holme O, Green S, Kuiper T, Marmo R, Omar M, Petruzziello L, Spada C, Zullo A, Dumonceau JM, European Society of Gastrointestinal Endoscopy. Bowel preparation for colonoscopy: European Society of Gastrointestinal Endoscopy (ESGE) guideline. Endoscopy. 2013;45(2):142–50. https://doi.org/10.1055/s-0032-1326186.
14. Committee ASoP, Saltzman JR, Cash BD, Pasha SF, Early DS, Muthusamy VR, Khashab MA, Chathadi KV, Fanelli RD, Chandrasekhara V, Lightdale JR, Fonkalsrud L, Shergill AK, Hwang JH, Decker GA, Jue TL, Sharaf R, Fisher DA, Evans JA, Foley K, Shaukat A, Eloubeidi MA, Faulx AL, Wang A, Acosta RD. Bowel preparation before colonoscopy. Gastrointest Endosc. 2015;81(4):781–94. https://doi.org/10.1016/j.gie.2014.09.048.
15. Gurudu SR, Ramirez FC, Harrison ME, Leighton JA, Crowell MD. Increased adenoma detection rate with system-wide implementation of a split-dose preparation for colonoscopy. Gastrointest Endosc. 2012;76(3):603–608 e601. https://doi.org/10.1016/j.gie.2012.04.456.
16. Clark BT, Rustagi T, Laine L. What level of bowel prep quality requires early repeat colonoscopy: systematic review and meta-analysis of the impact of preparation quality on adenoma detection rate. Am J Gastroenterol. 2014;109(11):1714–1723.; quiz 1724. https://doi.org/10.1038/ajg.2014.232.
17. Adler A, Wegscheider K, Lieberman D, Aminalai A, Aschenbeck J, Drossel R, Mayr M, Mross M, Scheel M, Schroder A, Gerber K, Stange G, Roll S, Gauger U, Wiedenmann B, Altenhofen L, Rosch T. Factors determining the quality of screening colonoscopy: a prospective study on adenoma detection rates, from 12,134 examinations (berlin colonoscopy project 3, BECOP-3). Gut. 2013;62(2):236–41. https://doi.org/10.1136/gutjnl-2011-300167.
18. Tholey DM, Shelton CE, Francis G, Anantharaman A, Frankel RA, Shah P, Coan A, Hegarty SE, Leiby BE, Kastenberg DM. Adenoma detection in excellent versus good bowel preparation for colonoscopy. J Clin Gastroenterol. 2015;49(4):313–9. https://doi.org/10.1097/MCG.0000000000000270.
19. Clark BT, Laine L. High-quality bowel preparation is required for detection of sessile serrated polyps. Clin Gastroenterol Hepatol. 2016;14(8):1155–62. https://doi.org/10.1016/j.cgh.2016.03.044.
20. Calderwood AH, Thompson KD, Schroy PC 3rd, Lieberman DA, Jacobson BC. Good is better than excellent: bowel preparation quality and adenoma detection rates. Gastrointest Endosc. 2015;81(3):691–699 e691. https://doi.org/10.1016/j.gie.2014.10.032.
21. Barclay RL, Vicari JJ, Doughty AS, Johanson JF, Greenlaw RL. Colonoscopic withdrawal times and adenoma detection during screening colonoscopy. N Engl J Med. 2006;355(24):2533–41. https://doi.org/10.1056/NEJMoa055498.
22. Jover R, Zapater P, Polania E, Bujanda L, Lanas A, Hermo JA, Cubiella J, Ono A, Gonzalez-Mendez Y, Peris A, Pellise M, Seoane A, Herreros-de-Tejada A, Ponce M, Marin-Gabriel JC, Chaparro M, Cacho G, Fernandez-Diez S, Arenas J, Sopena F, de Castro L, Vega-Villaamil P, Rodriguez-Soler M, Carballo F, Salas D, Morillas JD, Andreu M, Quintero E, Castells A, investigators Cs. Modifiable endoscopic factors that influence the adenoma detection rate in colorectal cancer screening colonoscopies. Gastrointest Endosc. 2013;77(3):381–389 e381. https://doi.org/10.1016/j.gie.2012.09.027.
23. Butterly L, Robinson CM, Anderson JC, Weiss JE, Goodrich M, Onega TL, Amos CI, Beach ML. Serrated and adenomatous polyp detection increases with longer withdrawal time: results from the New Hampshire colonoscopy registry. Am J Gastroenterol. 2014;109(3):417–26. https://doi.org/10.1038/ajg.2013.442.

24. Lee TJ, Blanks RG, Rees CJ, Wright KC, Nickerson C, Moss SM, Chilton A, Goddard AF, Patnick J, McNally RJ, Rutter MD. Longer mean colonoscopy withdrawal time is associated with increased adenoma detection: evidence from the bowel cancer screening programme in England. Endoscopy. 2013;45(1):20–6. https://doi.org/10.1055/s-0032-1325803.
25. Vavricka SR, Sulz MC, Degen L, Rechner R, Manz M, Biedermann L, Beglinger C, Peter S, Safroneeva E, Rogler G, Schoepfer AM. Monitoring colonoscopy withdrawal time significantly improves the adenoma detection rate and the performance of endoscopists. Endoscopy. 2016;48(3):256–62. https://doi.org/10.1055/s-0035-1569674.
26. Brenner H, Hoffmeister M, Arndt V, Stegmaier C, Altenhofen L, Haug U. Protection from right- and left-sided colorectal neoplasms after colonoscopy: population-based study. J Natl Cancer Inst. 2010;102(2):89–95. https://doi.org/10.1093/jnci/djp436.
27. Rex DK. How I approach Retroflexion and prevention of right-sided colon cancer following colonoscopy. Am J Gastroenterol. 2016;111(1):9–11. https://doi.org/10.1038/ajg.2015.385.
28. Hewett DG, Rex DK. Miss rate of right-sided colon examination during colonoscopy defined by retroflexion: an observational study. Gastrointest Endosc. 2011;74(2):246–52. https://doi.org/10.1016/j.gie.2011.04.005.
29. Kushnir VM, Oh YS, Hollander T, Chen CH, Sayuk GS, Davidson N, Mullady D, Murad FM, Sharabash NM, Ruettgers E, Dassopoulos T, Easler JJ, Gyawali CP, Edmundowicz SA, Early DS. Impact of retroflexion vs. second forward view examination of the right colon on adenoma detection: a comparison study. Am J Gastroenterol. 2015;110(3):415–22. https://doi.org/10.1038/ajg.2015.21.
30. Lee HS, Jeon SW, Park HY, Yeo SJ. Improved detection of right colon adenomas with additional retroflexion following two forward-view examinations: a prospective study. Endoscopy. 2016;49(4):334–41. https://doi.org/10.1055/s-0042-119401.
31. Triantafyllou K, Tziatzios G, Sioulas AD, Beintaris I, Gouloumi AR, Panayiotides IG, Dimitriadis GD. Diagnostic yield of scope retroflexion in the right colon: a prospective cohort study. Dig Liver Dis. 2016;48(2):176–81. https://doi.org/10.1016/j.dld.2015.11.024.
32. Leung FW. Water exchange may be superior to water immersion for colonoscopy. Clin Gastroenterol Hepatol. 2011;9(12):1012–4. https://doi.org/10.1016/j.cgh.2011.09.007.
33. Leung FW, Amato A, Ell C, Friedland S, Harker JO, Hsieh YH, Leung JW, Mann SK, Paggi S, Pohl J, Radaelli F, Ramirez FC, Siao-Salera R, Terruzzi V. Water-aided colonoscopy: a systematic review. Gastrointest Endosc. 2012;76(3):657–66. https://doi.org/10.1016/j.gie.2012.04.467.
34. Ramirez FC, Leung FW. A head-to-head comparison of the water vs. air method in patients undergoing screening colonoscopy. J Interv Gastroenterol. 2011;1(3):130–5. https://doi.org/10.4161/jig.1.3.18512.
35. Hafner S, Zolk K, Radaelli F, Otte J, Rabenstein T, Zolk O. Water infusion versus air insufflation for colonoscopy. Cochrane Database Syst Rev. 2015;5:CD009863. https://doi.org/10.1002/14651858.CD009863.pub2.
36. Hsieh YH, Koo M, Leung FW. A patient-blinded randomized, controlled trial comparing air insufflation, water immersion, and water exchange during minimally sedated colonoscopy. Am J Gastroenterol. 2014;109(9):1390–400. https://doi.org/10.1038/ajg.2014.126.
37. Cadoni S, Gallittu P, Sanna S, Fanari V, Porcedda ML, Erriu M, Leung FW. A two-center randomized controlled trial of water-aided colonoscopy versus air insufflation colonoscopy. Endoscopy. 2014;46(3):212–8. https://doi.org/10.1055/s-0033-1353604.
38. Hsieh YH, Tseng CW, Hu CT, Koo M, Leung FW. Prospective multicenter randomized controlled trial comparing adenoma detection rate in colonoscopy using water exchange, water immersion, and air insufflation. Gastrointest Endosc. 2016. https://doi.org/10.1016/j.gie.2016.12.005.
39. Xu L, Zhang Y, Song H, Wang W, Zhang S, Ding X. Nurse participation in colonoscopy observation versus the Colonoscopist alone for polyp and adenoma detection: a meta-analysis of randomized, controlled trials. Gastroenterol Res Pract. 2016;2016:7631981. https://doi.org/10.1155/2016/7631981.

40. Chalifoux SL, Rao DS, Wani SB, Sharma P, Bansal A, Gupta N, Rastogi A. Trainee participation and adenoma detection rates during screening colonoscopies. J Clin Gastroenterol. 2014;48(6):524–9. https://doi.org/10.1097/MCG.0000000000000022.
41. Buchner AM, Shahid MW, Heckman MG, Diehl NN, McNeil RB, Cleveland P, Gill KR, Schore A, Ghabril M, Raimondo M, Gross SA, Wallace MB. Trainee participation is associated with increased small adenoma detection. Gastrointest Endosc. 2011;73(6):1223–31. https://doi.org/10.1016/j.gie.2011.01.060.
42. Gianotti RJ, Oza SS, Tapper EB, Kothari D, Sheth SG. A longitudinal study of adenoma detection rate in gastroenterology fellowship training. Dig Dis Sci. 2016;61(10):2831–7. https://doi.org/10.1007/s10620-016-4228-9.
43. Harada Y, Hirasawa D, Fujita N, Noda Y, Kobayashi G, Ishida K, Yonechi M, Ito K, Suzuki T, Sugawara T, Horaguchi J, Takasawa O, Obana T, Oohira T, Onochi K, Kanno Y, Kuroha M, Iwai W. Impact of a transparent hood on the performance of total colonoscopy: a randomized controlled trial. Gastrointest Endosc. 2009;69(3 Pt 2):637–44. https://doi.org/10.1016/j.gie.2008.08.029.
44. Park SM, Lee SH, Shin KY, Heo J, Sung SH, Park SH, Choi SY, Lee DW, Park HG, Lee HS, Jeon SW, Kim SK, Jung MK. The cap-assisted technique enhances colonoscopy training: prospective randomized study of six trainees. Surg Endosc. 2012;26(10):2939–43. https://doi.org/10.1007/s00464-012-2288-2.
45. Rastogi A, Bansal A, Rao DS, Gupta N, Wani SB, Shipe T, Gaddam S, Singh V, Sharma P. Higher adenoma detection rates with cap-assisted colonoscopy: a randomised controlled trial. Gut. 2012;61(3):402–8. https://doi.org/10.1136/gutjnl-2011-300187.
46. Kim DJ, Kim HW, Park SB, Kang DH, Choi CW, Hong JB, Ji BH, Lee CS. Efficacy of cap-assisted colonoscopy according to lesion location and endoscopist training level. World J Gastroenterol. 2015;21(20):6261–70. https://doi.org/10.3748/wjg.v21.i20.6261.
47. Pohl H, Bensen SP, Toor A, Gordon SR, Levy LC, Berk B, Anderson PB, Anderson JC, Rothstein RI, MacKenzie TA, Robertson DJ. Cap-assisted colonoscopy and detection of adenomatous polyps (CAP) study: a randomized trial. Endoscopy. 2015;47(10):891–7. https://doi.org/10.1055/s-0034-1392261.
48. Lee YT, Lai LH, Hui AJ, Wong VW, Ching JY, Wong GL, Wu JC, Chan HL, Leung WK, Lau JY, Sung JJ, Chan FK. Efficacy of cap-assisted colonoscopy in comparison with regular colonoscopy: a randomized controlled trial. Am J Gastroenterol. 2009;104(1):41–6. https://doi.org/10.1038/ajg.2008.56.
49. Ng SC, Tsoi KK, Hirai HW, Lee YT, Wu JC, Sung JJ, Chan FK, Lau JY. The efficacy of cap-assisted colonoscopy in polyp detection and cecal intubation: a meta-analysis of randomized controlled trials. Am J Gastroenterol. 2012;107(8):1165–73. https://doi.org/10.1038/ajg.2012.135.
50. Tsiamoulos ZP, Saunders BP. A new accessory, endoscopic cuff, improves colonoscopic access for complex polyp resection and scar assessment in the sigmoid colon (with video). Gastrointest Endosc. 2012;76(6):1242–5. https://doi.org/10.1016/j.gie.2012.08.019.
51. Lenze F, Beyna T, Lenz P, Heinzow HS, Hengst K, Ullerich H. Endocuff-assisted colonoscopy: a new accessory to improve adenoma detection rate? Technical aspects and first clinical experiences. Endoscopy. 2014;46(7):610–4. https://doi.org/10.1055/s-0034-1365446.
52. Biecker E, Floer M, Heinecke A, Strobel P, Bohme R, Schepke M, Meister T. Novel endocuff-assisted colonoscopy significantly increases the polyp detection rate: a randomized controlled trial. J Clin Gastroenterol. 2015;49(5):413–8. https://doi.org/10.1097/MCG.0000000000000166.
53. Floer M, Biecker E, Fitzlaff R, Roming H, Ameis D, Heinecke A, Kunsch S, Ellenrieder V, Strobel P, Schepke M, Meister T. Higher adenoma detection rates with endocuff-assisted colonoscopy - a randomized controlled multicenter trial. PLoS One. 2014;9(12):e114267. https://doi.org/10.1371/journal.pone.0114267.
54. van Doorn SC, van der Vlugt M, Depla A, Wientjes CA, Mallant-Hent RC, Siersema PD, Tytgat K, Tuynman H, Kuiken SD, Houben G, Stokkers P, Moons L, Bossuyt P, Fockens P, Mundt MW, Dekker E. Adenoma detection with Endocuff colonoscopy versus conventional

colonoscopy: a multicentre randomised controlled trial. Gut. 2015;66(3):438–45. https://doi. org/10.1136/gutjnl-2015-310097.

55. Chin M, Karnes W, Jamal MM, Lee JG, Lee R, Samarasena J, Bechtold ML, Nguyen DL. Use of the Endocuff during routine colonoscopy examination improves adenoma detection: a meta-analysis. World J Gastroenterol. 2016;22(43):9642–9. https://doi.org/10.3748/wjg.v22. i43.9642.

56. Triantafyllou K, Polymeros D, Apostolopoulos P, Brandao C, Gkolfakis P, Repici A, Papanikolaou IS, Dinis-Ribeiro M, Alexandrakis G, Hassan C. Endocuff-assisted colonoscopy outperforms conventional colonoscopy to detect missed-adenomas: european multicenter, randomized, back-to-back study. United European Gastroenterol J. 2016;2 Suppl 1.

57. Bevan R, Ngu WS, Saunders BP, Tsiamoulos Z, Bassett P, Hoare Z, Rees CJ. The ADENOMA study. Accuracy of detection using Endocuff vision optimization of mucosal abnormalities: study protocol for randomized controlled trial. Endosc Int Open. 2016;4(2):E205–12. https:// doi.org/10.1055/s-0041-107900.

58. Dik VK, Gralnek IM, Segol O, Suissa A, Belderbos TD, Moons LM, Segev M, Domanov S, Rex DK, Siersema PD. Multicenter, randomized, tandem evaluation of EndoRings colonoscopy--results of the CLEVER study. Endoscopy. 2015;47(12):1151–8. https://doi.org/10.105 5/s-0034-1392421.

59. Gralnek IM, Suissa A, Domanov S. Safety and efficacy of a novel balloon colonoscope: a prospective cohort study. Endoscopy. 2014;46(10):883–7. https://doi.org/10.105 5/s-0034-1377968.

60. Halpern Z, Gross SA, Gralnek IM, Shpak B, Pochapin M, Hoffman A, Mizrahi M, Rochberger YS, Moshkowitz M, Santo E, Melhem A, Grinshpon R, Pfefer J, Kiesslich R. Comparison of adenoma detection and miss rates between a novel balloon colonoscope and standard colonoscopy: a randomized tandem study. Endoscopy. 2015;47(4):301. https://doi.org/10.105 5/s-0034-1391894.

61. Rubin M, Lurie L, Bose K, Kim SH. Expanding the view of a standard colonoscope with the third eye panoramic cap. World J Gastroenterol. 2015;21(37):10683–7. https://doi. org/10.3748/wjg.v21.i37.10683.

62. Gralnek IM, Segol O, Suissa A, Siersema PD, Carr-Locke DL, Halpern Z, Santo E, Domanov S. A prospective cohort study evaluating a novel colonoscopy platform featuring full-spectrum endoscopy. Endoscopy. 2013;45(9):697–702. https://doi.org/10.1055/s-0033-1344395.

63. Gralnek IM, Siersema PD, Halpern Z, Segol O, Melhem A, Suissa A, Santo E, Sloyer A, Fenster J, Moons LM, Dik VK, D'Agostino RB Jr, Rex DK. Standard forward-viewing colonoscopy versus full-spectrum endoscopy: an international, multicentre, randomised, tandem colonoscopy trial. Lancet Oncol. 2014;15(3):353–60. https://doi.org/10.1016/ S1470-2045(14)70020-8.

64. Papanikolaou IS, Apostolopoulos P, Tziatzios G, Vlachou E, Sioulas AD, Polymeros D, Karameris A, Panayiotides I, Alexandrakis G, Dimitriadis GD, Triantafyllou K. Lower adenoma miss rate with FUSE vs. conventional colonoscopy with proximal retroflexion: a randomized back-to-back trial. Endoscopy. 2017;49(5):468–75. https://doi.org/10.1055/s-0042-124415.

65. Hassan C, Senore C, Radaelli F, De Pretis G, Sassatelli R, Arrigoni A, Manes G, Amato A, Anderloni A, Armelao F, Mondardini A, Spada C, Omazzi B, Cavina M, Miori G, Campanale C, Sereni G, Segnan N, Repici A. Full-spectrum (FUSE) versus standard forward-viewing colonoscopy in an organised colorectal cancer screening programme. Gut. 2016:gutjnl-2016-311906. https://doi.org/10.1136/gutjnl-2016-311906.

66. van den Broek FJ, Kuiper T, Dekker E, Zwinderman AH, Fockens P, Reitsma JB. Study designs to compare new colonoscopic techniques: clinical considerations, data analysis, and sample size calculations. Endoscopy. 2013;45(11):922–7. https://doi.org/10.1055/s-0033-1344434.

67. Uraoka T, Tanaka S, Oka S, Matsuda T, Saito Y, Moriyama T, Higashi R, Matsumoto T. Feasibility of a novel colonoscope with extra-wide angle of view: a clinical study. Endoscopy. 2015;47(5):444–8. https://doi.org/10.1055/s-0034-1390870.

Non-polypoid Colorectal Neoplasms: Characteristics and Endoscopic Management

3

Maria Antonia Bianco, Cristina Bucci, and Fabiana Zingone

3.1 Chapter

The progress in endoscopy, from forceps biopsy to advanced optical diagnosis, has led to several changes in the clinical and pathological approach of colorectal tumors. Nowadays, advanced optical diagnosis offers the possibility to spot irregular, elevated, or depressed mucosal areas or alterations of the vascular pattern (lack or increase thereof), making it possible to obtain an easier identification and a better characterization of preneoplastic lesions. It is now possible to correlate the glandular and vascular architecture to the histological pattern, so as to be able to understand in advance the degree of neoplastic infiltration and plan the correct therapeutic approach (e.g., endoscopic resection vs. surgical resection).

Endoscopic detection and resection of superficial colon lesions are now considered the gold standard for colorectal cancer (CRC) prevention. In fact, it is well known that CRC arises from precancerous (adenomatous) lesions mainly through the "adenoma-carcinoma sequence" and that removing adenomatous polyps can alter this pathway. Moreover, in recent years a different pathway through the sessile serrated adenoma/polyp (SSA/P) sequence has also been recognized as a precursor of colorectal cancer, but spotting and classification of these lesions have proved more difficult to perform, compared to the traditional adenomas [1, 2].

An explicit recognition goes together with a correct classification of the lesions. According to the most accepted classification, the Paris classification, mucosal lesions are categorized as protruding or polypoid ($\geq$2.5 mm above the mucosal layer or type I), non-protruding or non-polypoid (<2.5 mm above the mucosal layer or type II) and excavated (type III) [3, 4]. Polypoid types are subdivided into pedunculated (0-Ip), sessile (0-Is), or mixed (0-Isp) while non-polypoid as slightly elevated (0-IIa),

M.A. Bianco (✉) • C. Bucci • F. Zingone
Gastrointestinal Unit, ASL Na3 SUD, Torre del Greco, Naples, Italy
e-mail: biancoendo@gmail.com

© Springer International Publishing AG 2018
A. Facciorusso, N. Muscatiello (eds.), *Colon Polypectomy*,
https://doi.org/10.1007/978-3-319-59457-6_3

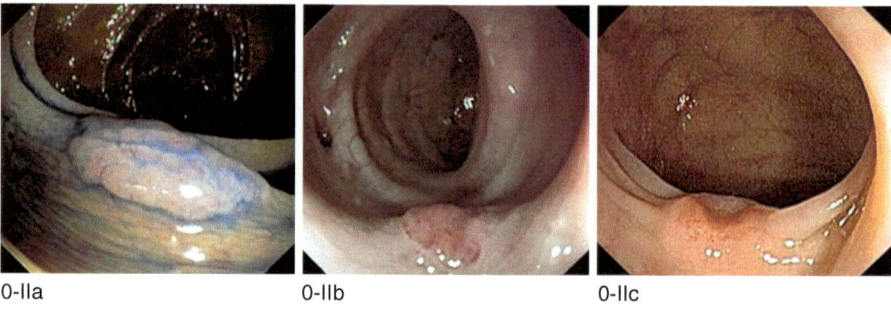

0-IIa   0-IIb   0-IIc

Fig. 3.1 Non-polypoid lesions according to the Paris classification

flat (0-IIb), or slightly depressed (0-IIc) [3, 4] (Fig. 3.1). The threshold of 2.5 mm, which corresponds to the height of a closed biopsy forceps, is entirely arbitrary and is one of the pitfalls for nonexpert endoscopists. For example, only recently the validity and reproducibility of the Paris classification have been assessed, exposing a barely moderate intra-observer pre- and post-digital training agreement (Fleiss kappa of 0.42 and a mean pairwise agreement of 67%) with the lower concordance in the proportion of lesions assessed as "flat" [5]. Also, slightly elevated (0-IIa) lesions are often misclassified as sessile (0-Is), as demonstrated by the histopathological revision of 933 adenomas found in the National Polyp Study, initially classified as sessile. Of those, 474 were reclassified as flat adenomas [6].

The laterally spreading tumor (LST), firstly recognized by Kudo as a subtype of non-polypoid lesions [7], is a large (>10 mm) flat superficial lesion that grows laterally along the surface of the colon, in opposition to polypoid (upward growth) or flat lesions (downward growth). LST is divided into the granular (LST-G) and non-granular type (LST-NG), according to the presence/absence of conglomerates of nodules [3, 4]. The previous literature showed a different distribution of LST along the colon, being the LST-G type the most frequent macroscopic finding in the rectum, whereas LST-NG was detected more frequently in the colon. Moreover, the LSTs in the rectum were significantly larger and with a higher incidence of high-grade dysplasia than those found in the colon [8, 9].

Kudo et al. showed the importance of non-polypoid lesions (NPL) for the first time in the 1990s in Japan [10, 11]. These eventually became relatively common also in Western countries, with a prevalence ranging from 5 to 36% [12, 13]. In 2010, a large Italian multicenter study that analyzed data from 27.400 colonoscopies confirmed that their prevalence was at 5.3% and showed that NPLs accounted for 25.9% of all neoplasms detected during endoscopic examination. Authors also found that NPLs were more common in the right colon compared to polypoid lesions (48.9% vs. 31.7%) and that the risk of advanced histology was not related to morphology (NPL vs. polypoid), except for depressed subtypes ($p < 0.001$) [13].

Generally speaking, whether polypoid (e.g., protruding) and non-polypoid (e.g., flat) lesions should be regarded as different endoscopic entities is still a matter of debate [14]. Compared to polypoid lesions, NPLs are more frequently located in the right colon and in older patients. Further, they carry a higher risk of deeper invasions (only for depressed subtype) and require dedicated endoscopic techniques to be removed endoscopically [15]. In a recent retrospective study, the authors analyzed 5.768 colonoscopies to detect the clinical characteristics of post-colonoscopy advanced neoplasms within 5.5 years from the primary colonoscopy. They found that the incidence of NPL in the post-colonoscopy advanced neoplasms (25.6%, 41/160) was statistically higher than that in the primary lesions (12.3%, 67/545, $p < 0.001$), suggesting that endoscopists should reserve extra attention to non-polypoid, right-sided lesions [16]. Moreover, a recent multicenter retrospective study found that supplementary factors can influence the recognition of flat lesions. In the multivariate analysis the authors showed that older age, presence of concomitant protruding adenomas, poor bowel preparation, smaller adenoma size, location in the right colon, insufficient experience of the endoscopists, and withdrawal time < 6 min were associated with an increased missing rate for flat adenomas [17].

Lesions suitable for endoscopic resection are those confined to the mucosa (or superficial layer of submucosa in selected cases), whereas deeper invasion makes endoscopic therapy infeasible [18].

In the early 1990s, Kikuchi et al. [19] classified the submucosal invasion into three levels: Sm1, invasion into the upper third of the submucosa; Sm2, invasion into the middle third of the submucosa; and Sm3, invasion into the lower third of the submucosa. This classification, together with the Haggitt classification, has been shown to correlate with the risk of lymphonode metastasis, being 1–3% in Sm1 lesions, 8% in Sm2 lesions, and 23% in Sm3 lesions [20].

Hence, it is essential to learn how to differentiate benign lesions from cancers before undertaking endoscopic resections [21]. Simple random biopsies of flat lesions should be avoided because biopsies may miss cancer in a large polyp or a flat lesion; also, biopsies may cause submucosal fibrosis and preclude safe and complete resections in the future. The effects of prior biopsy sampling on endoscopic resection have been recently evaluated via analyses of 132 non-pedunculated colorectal lesions ≥20 mm: 46 lesions without any prior manipulation, 44 with only prior biopsy sampling, and 42 with prior advanced manipulation, including tattoo and/or snare sampling. The en bloc resection rate was observed in 34.8% of cases for non-manipulated lesions, in 15.9% for lesions with prior biopsy sampling, and in 4.8% for lesions with prior advanced manipulation ($p = 0.001$). Complete endoscopic resection without the need for ablation of visible residual was performed in 93.5% of the non-manipulated lesions, 68.2% of lesions with prior biopsy sampling, and 50% of lesions with prior advanced manipulation ($p < 0.001$). Recurrence rates were 7.7, 40.7, and 53.8% in the three groups ($p = 0.001$) [22].

In flat lesions, some endoscopic signs may be regarded as in vivo predictors of deeper submucosal invasion (Sm 2/3), such as expansive appearance, deep depression surface, irregular bottom of depression surface, folds converging toward the tumor, and nodule >10 mm [23].

Furthermore, the diffusion of *advanced endoscopy techniques* can help to identify invasive lesions with a specificity higher than 98%, avoiding useless endoscopy resections and giving instead immediate indication to surgery [23–28]. In fact, the use of advanced optical techniques has been shown to be an effective adjunct to discriminate among hyperplasic lesions, adenomas with dysplasia, and invasive cancer. The rationale behind the widespread use of advanced imaging is its ability to correctly classify superficial lesions according to their risk of mucosal/submucosal invasion and to avoid the risk of over- or under-endoscopic treatment.

Chromoendoscopy made its first appearance in the literature in the 1970s. This technique, based on the use of contrast dyes to improve the detection of mucosal abnormalities, was additionally implemented by the use of magnifying endoscopy (or *magnifying chromoendoscopy*). This adjustable focusing mechanism enlarges the image from 1.5× to 150× in order to visualize fine details of mucosal surface pattern and vascular architecture. Kudo et al. in 1996 first described the application of magnified endoscopy to classified colorectal polyps according to their appearance, structure, and staining patterns by studying the orifices of the colonic crypts "pit" to distinguish neoplastic and non-neoplastic polyps [29]. Additionally, revisions of the original Kudo classification subclassified the type V pit pattern into type V_i (irregular) and type V_N (nonstructural), as type V_I has been shown to be an index of adenoma with severe dysplasia or Sm1 carcinoma, while type V_N is an indicator of invasion more than Sm1 [30, 31] or, according to the criteria of Nagata et al., on the basis of the appearance of the V_N pit pattern into three types (A–C) with regard to the invasion depth [32]. To date, several trials have demonstrated that Kudo's pit pattern classification (Fig. 3.2) is a highly accurate diagnostic method to differentiate neoplastic from non-neoplastic lesions. This was confirmed by a recent meta-analysis showing that Kudo's classification has a pooled sensitivity of 89.0 and 85.7% specificity for the diagnosis of colorectal neoplastic polyps [33, 34].

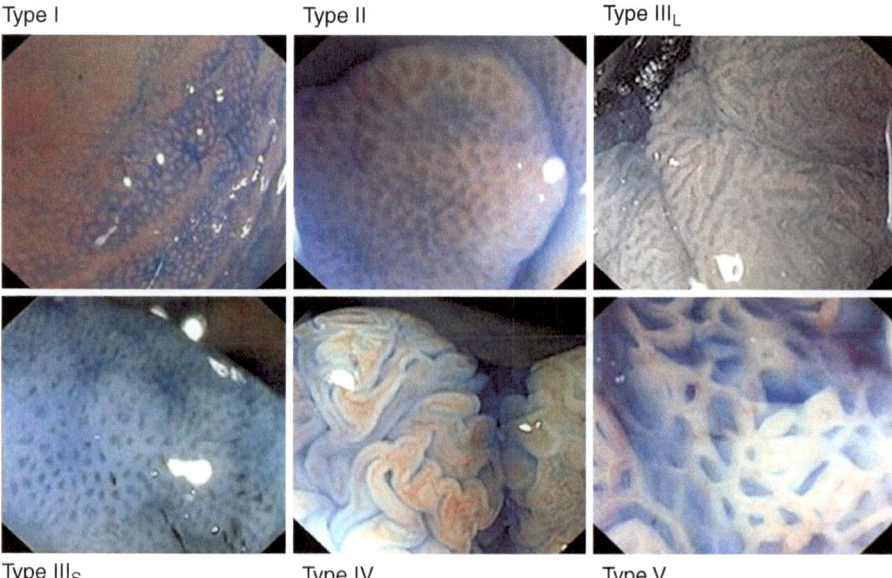

Fig. 3.2 Pit pattern according to the Kudo classification

Also, the efficacy of magnification chromoendoscopy was specifically tested for the endoscopic assessment of submucosal invasion in flat and depressed colorectal lesions in different clinical trials, showing a 97% sensitivity in predicting Sm2 invasion but with a lower overall specificity (50%) [25] and a PPV of 79% and a NPV of 98% [26], confirming that the routine use of chromoendoscopy in routine practice is still disputable [35, 36].

Narrowband imaging (NBI), developed by Sano et al. in 1999, is a high-resolution endoscopic technique that enhances the fine structure of the mucosal surface without the use of dyes [37]. Unlike chromoendoscopy that requires experience, is time-consuming, and is expensive, NBI and other digital chromoendoscopy techniques (e.g., FICE and I-Scan) are computed virtual chromoendoscopies that allow, via a touch-button technology, to obtain a more definite visualization of gastrointestinal superficial lesions. Narrowband imaging (NBI; Olympus Inc., Hauppauge, NY, USA), flexible spectral imaging color enhancement (FICE; Fujinon Inc., Saitama, Japan), and I-Scan (Pentax Inc., Tokyo, Japan) are the most widely used and commercially available methods.

NBI technology uses short-wave blue and green light sources and blocks red wavelengths, improving the visualization of mucosal vessels, which are frequently altered in form, density, and size in colorectal lesions [38]. Also, if employed with zoom endoscopy, it enables the analysis of pit pattern subtypes. The use of NBI technique has validated different classifications. The most widely used classification by Western endoscopists is the NICE classification, based on the color, vessels, and surface pattern on endoscopy [39, 40] (Fig. 3.3). In Japan, beginning with the Sano classification, which was the first published NBI magnifying endoscopic classification [41, 42], many other ones were validated, such as the Hiroshima and Showa classifications, and published in 2008 and 2009, respectively. The latter added the characteristics of the surface pattern to the vascular findings on NBI

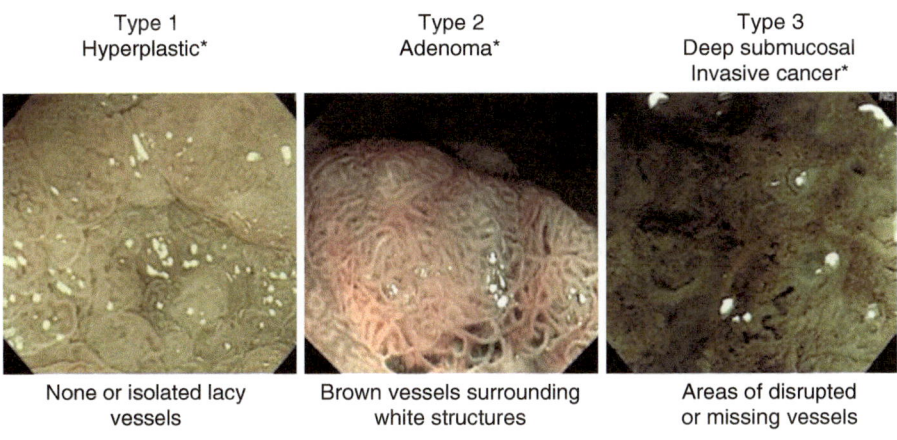

Type 1 Hyperplastic*	Type 2 Adenoma*	Type 3 Deep submucosal Invasive cancer*
None or isolated lacy vessels	Brown vessels surrounding white structures	Areas of disrupted or missing vessels

*most likely pathology

Fig. 3.3 Endoscopy findings of NICE classification

magnifying endoscopy. To unify and simplify the use of different scales, in 2009 a simple NBI endoscopic classification of colorectal tumors, called the JNET classification, was created [43].

However, regardless of the classification used, mixed results have been associated with the use of NBI in the colon for adenoma detection. In a meta-analysis in 2012, Pasha et al. showed no significant difference between the use of high-definition NBI (HD-NBI) and high-definition white light endoscopy (HD-WLE) in patients undergoing screening/surveillance colonoscopy with regard to the detection of any-size adenomas, adenomas smaller than 10 mm, or flat adenomas nor in the miss rate of colon polyps or adenomas [44]. Interestingly, a subsequent trial by Adler et al. suggested that NBI does not increase the adenoma detection rate per se, but it could induce a "learning effect" in detecting subtle lesions with traditional WLE, since detection improved in the WLE group as the study progressed [45]. Conversely, NBI appears to be more useful in the characterization of neoplastic superficial lesions with an overall sensitivity of 91.0%, specificity of 82.6%, and NPVs exceeding 90% when 60% or less of all polyps were neoplastic. Noteworthy is the fact that the surveillance intervals based on NBI endoscopic diagnosis agreed with pathology in 92.6% of patients [46].

Unlike NBI, which uses physical filters, *FICE and I-Scan* are based on a software technology that achieves vascular enhancement with the use of postprocessor technology. Fewer trials have been published with the aim of validating these technologies, and based on those published they do not seem to improve the overall adenoma detection rate (ADR) nor the detection of subtypes of adenomas, although they appear as reasonably accurate for characterization of colorectal lesions [47, 48].

Finally, advanced endoscopy techniques include the *confocal laser endomicroscopy (CLE)*, a novel optical biopsy procedure designed to provide in vivo histology and facilitate diagnosis with real-time intervention, thus avoiding biopsy samples [49]. A meta-analysis has assessed the accuracy of CLE in the in vivo prediction of colorectal lesions histology. Results showed that the weighted and total pooled result for sensitivity was 81%, whereas it was 88% for specificity. As a consequence, CLE could be regarded as a valuable in vivo endoscopic method to distinguish neoplastic from nonneoplastic lesions [50].

When the endoscopy resection is considered possible, the dimensional criteria of the lesion and the operator's expertise should define which type of technique to use: *endoscopic mucosal resection (EMR) or endoscopic submucosal dissection (ESD)*. Lesions smaller than 2 cm can be safely removed by EMR en bloc, while larger lesions should be removed by EMR piecemeal or by ESD en bloc. In fact, although ESD has a longer procedure time and a higher perforation rate for lesion ≥ 20 mm, its use gives a higher rate of en bloc resection, compared with EMR [51, 52].

A meta-analysis comparing ESD and EMR (six retrospective case-control studies, four in Japan, and two in South Korea, for a total of 1642 lesions) described better results with ESD compared to EMR in term of en bloc resection [OR = 7.94 (95%CI, 3.96–15.91)], local recurrence [OR = 0.09 (95%CI, 0.04–0.19)], and histological (R0) resection [OR = 1.65 (95%CI, 0.29–9.30)], yielding no difference in procedure-related complication [OR = 1.59 (95%CI, 0.92–2.73)] [53].

However, the EMR piecemeal technique can still be considered a valid choice for large lesions resection. A multicenter Australian prospective study showed that, following colonic wide-field EMR, early recurrent/residual adenoma occurred in 16%, and it was usually unifocal and diminutive, whereas late recurrence occurred in 4%. Overall, recurrence was managed endoscopically in 93% of cases. Risk factors for recurrence were lesions size >40 mm, use of argon plasma coagulation, and intra-procedural bleeding [54].

Repici et al. performed a systematic review including a total of 22 studies (20 Asian, 2 European), providing data on 2841 ESD-treated lesions. A complete resection was obtained in 88% considering the Asian studies, but only in 65% considering the two European studies, showing an extreme heterogeneity in the use and expertise of the ESD in Eastern and Western countries [55].

In a multicenter prospective Italian study, Cipolletta et al. found that in 385 lesions larger than 25 mm, 95.6% of them were removed using the EMR piecemeal technique and only a 4.4% using ESD. A complete resection was obtained in 85.8% of cases and a 12-month residual/recurrence in 6.5% of cases [56].

We can consider a radical intervention when the margins are free from lesions (R0), and we should receive the following information by the histological report [57–59]:

1. Degree of submucosal infiltration (greater or lesser than 1000 μm)
2. Lymphatic or hematic spread (V-L)
3. Degree of differentiation (well, moderately or poorly differentiated)
4. Presence of ulceration
5. Budding grade

In conclusion, non-polypoid lesions are common findings during routine colonoscopies, but their identification can be more challenging compared to polypoid lesions and therefore should be carefully searched. Once detected, advanced endoscopy techniques, such as chromoendoscopy or NBI, should be routinely employed to better define these lesions in terms of deep invasion and to plan the most correct endoscopic therapeutic approach.

References

1. Rex DK, Ahnen DJ, Baron JA, Batts KP, Burke CA, Burt RW, et al. Serrated lesions of the colorectum: review and recommendations from an expert panel. Am J Gastroenterol. 2012;107(9):1315–29. quiz 4, 30.
2. Okamoto K, Kitamura S, Kimura T, Nakagawa T, Sogabe M, Miyamoto H, et al. Clinicopathological characteristics of serrated polyps as precursors to colorectal cancer: current status and management. J Gastroenterol Hepatol. 2017;32(2):358–67.
3. The Paris endoscopic classification of superficial neoplastic lesions: esophagus, stomach, and colon: November 30 to December 1, 2002. Gastrointest Endosc. 2003;58(6 Suppl):S3–43.
4. Update on the paris classification of superficial neoplastic lesions in the digestive tract. Endoscopy. 2005;37(6):570–8.
5. Gupta S. Trouble in Paris (classification): polyp morphology is in the eye of the beholder. Am J Gastroenterol. 2015;110(1):188–91.

6. O'Brien MJ, Winawer SJ, Zauber AG, Bushey MT, Sternberg SS, Gottlieb LS, et al. Flat adenomas in the National Polyp Study: is there increased risk for high-grade dysplasia initially or during surveillance? Clin Gastroenterol Hepatol. 2004;2(10):905–11.
7. Kudo S. Early colorectal cancer: detection of depressed types of colorectal carcinoma. Tokyo: Igaku-Shoin Ltd; 1996.
8. Konishi K, Fujii T, Boku N, Kato S, Koba I, Ohtsu A, et al. Clinicopathological differences between colonic and rectal carcinomas: are they based on the same mechanism of carcinogenesis? Gut. 1999;45(6):818–21.
9. Miyamoto H, Ikematsu H, Fujii S, Osera S, Odagaki T, Oono Y, et al. Clinicopathological differences of laterally spreading tumors arising in the colon and rectum. Int J Color Dis. 2014;29(9):1069–75.
10. Kudo S, Kashida H, Nakajima T, Tamura S, Nakajo K. Endoscopic diagnosis and treatment of early colorectal cancer. World J Surg. 1997;21(7):694–701.
11. Kudo S. Endoscopic mucosal resection of flat and depressed types of early colorectal cancer. Endoscopy. 1993;25(7):455–61.
12. Rembacken BJ, Fujii T, Cairns A, Dixon MF, Yoshida S, Chalmers DM, et al. Flat and depressed colonic neoplasms: a prospective study of 1000 colonoscopies in the UK. Lancet. 2000;355(9211):1211–4.
13. Bianco MA, Cipolletta L, Rotondano G, Buffoli F, Gizzi G, Tessari F, et al. Prevalence of nonpolypoid colorectal neoplasia: an Italian multicenter observational study. Endoscopy. 2010;42(4):279–85.
14. Lau PC, Sung JJ. Flat adenoma in colon: two decades of debate. J Dig Dis. 2010;11(4):201–7.
15. Park DH, Kim HS, Kim WH, Kim TI, Kim YH, Park DI, et al. Clinicopathologic characteristics and malignant potential of colorectal flat neoplasia compared with that of polypoid neoplasia. Dis Colon Rectum. 2008;51(1):43–9. Discussion 9.
16. Kawamura T, Uno K, Tanaka K, Ueda Y, Sakiyama N, Nishida K, et al. Morphological characteristics and location of missed, advanced colorectal neoplasms after colonoscopy. J Med Investig. 2016;63(3–4):163–70.
17. Xiang L, Zhan Q, Zhao XH, Wang YD, An SL, Xu YZ, et al. Risk factors associated with missed colorectal flat adenoma: a multicenter retrospective tandem colonoscopy study. World J Gastroenterol. 2014;20(31):10927–37.
18. Facciorusso A, Antonino M, Di Maso M, Barone M, Muscatiello N. Non-polypoid colorectal neoplasms: classification, therapy and follow-up. World J Gastroenterol. 2015;21(17):5149–57.
19. Kikuchi R, Takano M, Takagi K, Fujimoto N, Nozaki R, Fujiyoshi T, et al. Management of early invasive colorectal cancer. Risk of recurrence and clinical guidelines. Dis Colon Rectum. 1995;38(12):1286–95.
20. Tytherleigh MG, Warren BF, Mortensen NJ. Management of early rectal cancer. Br J Surg. 2008;95(4):409–23.
21. Tanaka S, Kashida H, Saito Y, Yahagi N, Yamano H, Saito S, et al. JGES guidelines for colorectal endoscopic submucosal dissection/endoscopic mucosal resection. Dig Endosc. 2015;27(4):417–34.
22. Kim HG, Thosani N, Banerjee S, Chen A, Friedland S. Effect of prior biopsy sampling, tattoo placement, and snare sampling on endoscopic resection of large nonpedunculated colorectal lesions. Gastrointest Endosc. 2015;81(1):204–13.
23. Saitoh Y, Obara T, Watari J, Nomura M, Taruishi M, Orii Y, et al. Invasion depth diagnosis of depressed type early colorectal cancers by combined use of videoendoscopy and chromoendoscopy. Gastrointest Endosc. 1998;48(4):362–70.
24. Kaltenbach T, Soetikno R. Image-enhanced endoscopy is critical in the detection, diagnosis, and treatment of non-polypoid colorectal neoplasms. Gastrointest Endosc Clin N Am. 2010;20(3):471–85.
25. Hurlstone DP, Cross SS, Adam I, Shorthouse AJ, Brown S, Sanders DS, et al. Endoscopic morphological anticipation of submucosal invasion in flat and depressed colorectal lesions: clinical implications and subtype analysis of the kudo type V pit pattern using high-magnification-chromoscopic colonoscopy. Color Dis. 2004;6(5):369–75.

26. Bianco MA, Rotondano G, Marmo R, Garofano ML, Piscopo R, de Gregorio A, et al. Predictive value of magnification chromoendoscopy for diagnosing invasive neoplasia in nonpolypoid colorectal lesions and stratifying patients for endoscopic resection or surgery. Endoscopy. 2006;38(5):470–6.
27. Asge Technology Committee, Song LM, Adler DG, Conway JD, Diehl DL, Farraye FA, et al. Narrow band imaging and multiband imaging. Gastrointest Endosc. 2008;67(4):581–9.
28. Asge Technology Committee, Kwon RS, Adler DG, Chand B, Conway JD, Diehl DL, et al. High-resolution and high-magnification endoscopes. Gastrointest Endosc. 2009;69(3 Pt 1):399–407.
29. Kudo S, Tamura S, Nakajima T, Yamano H, Kusaka H, Watanabe H. Diagnosis of colorectal tumorous lesions by magnifying endoscopy. Gastrointest Endosc. 1996;44(1):8–14.
30. Kudo S, Rubio CA, Teixeira CR, Kashida H, Kogure E. Pit pattern in colorectal neoplasia: endoscopic magnifying view. Endoscopy. 2001;33(4):367–73.
31. Fujii T, Hasegawa RT, Saitoh Y, Fleischer D, Saito Y, Sano Y, et al. Chromoscopy during colonoscopy. Endoscopy. 2001;33(12):1036–41.
32. Nagata S, Tanaka S, Haruma K, Yoshihara M, Sumii K, Kajiyama G, et al. Pit pattern diagnosis of early colorectal carcinoma by magnifying colonoscopy: clinical and histological implications. Int J Oncol. 2000;16(5):927–34.
33. Li M, Ali SM, Umm-a-OmarahGilani S, Liu J, Li YQ, Zuo XL. Kudo's pit pattern classification for colorectal neoplasms: a meta-analysis. World J Gastroenterol. 2014;20(35):12649–56.
34. Fu KI, Sano Y, Kato S, Fujii T, Nagashima F, Yoshino T, et al. Chromoendoscopy using indigo carmine dye spraying with magnifying observation is the most reliable method for differential diagnosis between non-neoplastic and neoplastic colorectal lesions: a prospective study. Endoscopy. 2004;36(12):1089–93.
35. Le Rhun M, Coron E, Parlier D, Nguyen JM, Canard JM, Alamdari A, et al. High resolution colonoscopy with chromoscopy versus standard colonoscopy for the detection of colonic neoplasia: a randomized study. Clin GastroenterolHepatol. 2006;4(3):349–54.
36. Brown SR, Baraza W, Din S, Riley S. Chromoscopy versus conventional endoscopy for the detection of polyps in the colon and rectum. Cochrane Database Syst Rev. 2016;4:CD006439.
37. Sano Y. New diagnostic method based on color imaging using narrow-band imaging (NBI) system for gastrointestinal tract. Gastrointest Endosc. 2001;53:AB125.
38. Hurlstone DP. The detection of flat and depressed colorectal lesions: which endoscopic imaging approach? Gastroenterology. 2008;135(2):338–43.
39. Hewett DG, Kaltenbach T, Sano Y, Tanaka S, Saunders BP, Ponchon T, et al. Validation of a simple classification system for endoscopic diagnosis of small colorectal polyps using narrow-band imaging. Gastroenterology. 2012;143(3):599–607 e1.
40. Hayashi N, Tanaka S, Hewett DG, Kaltenbach TR, Sano Y, Ponchon T, et al. Endoscopic prediction of deep submucosal invasive carcinoma: validation of the narrow-band imaging international colorectal endoscopic (NICE) classification. Gastrointest Endosc. 2013;78(4):625–32.
41. Machida H, Sano Y, Hamamoto Y, Muto M, Kozu T, Tajiri H, et al. Narrow-band imaging in the diagnosis of colorectal mucosal lesions: a pilot study. Endoscopy. 2004;36(12):1094–8.
42. Sano Y, Horimatsu T, Fu KI, Katagiri A, Muto M, Ishikawa H. Magnifying observation of microvascular architecture of colorectal lesions using a narrow-band imaging system. Dig Endosc. 2006;18(s1):S44–51.
43. Sumimoto K, Tanaka S, Shigita K, Hirano D, Tamaru Y, Ninomiya Y, et al. Clinical impact and characteristics of the narrow-band imaging magnifying endoscopic classification of colorectal tumors proposed by the Japan NBI Expert Team. Gastrointest Endosc. 2017;85(4):816–21.
44. Pasha SF, Leighton JA, Das A, Harrison ME, Gurudu SR, Ramirez FC, et al. Comparison of the yield and miss rate of narrow band imaging and white light endoscopy in patients undergoing screening or surveillance colonoscopy: a meta-analysis. Am J Gastroenterol. 2012;107(3):363–70.
45. Adler A, Pohl H, Papanikolaou IS, Abou-Rebyeh H, Schachschal G, Veltzke-Schlieker W, et al. A prospective randomised study on narrow-band imaging versus conventional

colonoscopy for adenoma detection: does narrow-band imaging induce a learning effect? Gut. 2008;57(1):59–64.

46. McGill SK, Evangelou E, Ioannidis JP, Soetikno RM, Kaltenbach T. Narrow band imaging to differentiate neoplastic and non-neoplastic colorectal polyps in real time: a meta-analysis of diagnostic operating characteristics. Gut. 2013;62(12):1704–13.

47. Chung SJ, Kim D, Song JH, Park MJ, Kim YS, Kim JS, et al. Efficacy of computed virtual chromoendoscopy on colorectal cancer screening: a prospective, randomized, back-to-back trial of Fuji intelligent color enhancement versus conventional colonoscopy to compare adenoma miss rates. Gastrointest Endosc. 2010;72(1):136–42.

48. Kim YS, Kim D, Chung SJ, Park MJ, Shin CS, Cho SH, et al. Differentiating small polyp histologies using real-time screening colonoscopy with Fuji intelligent color enhancement. Clin Gastroenterol Hepatol. 2011;9(9):744–9. e1.

49. Kiesslich R, Goetz M, Vieth M, Galle PR, Neurath MF. Confocal laser endomicroscopy. Gastrointest Endosc Clin N Am. 2005;15(4):715–31.

50. Dong YY, Li YQ, Yu YB, Liu J, Li M, Luan XR. Meta-analysis of confocal laser endomicroscopy for the detection of colorectal neoplasia. Color Dis. 2013;15(9):e488–95.

51. Saito Y, Fukuzawa M, Matsuda T, Fukunaga S, Sakamoto T, Uraoka T, et al. Clinical outcome of endoscopic submucosal dissection versus endoscopic mucosal resection of large colorectal tumors as determined by curative resection. Surg Endosc. 2010;24(2):343–52.

52. Lee EJ, Lee JB, Lee SH, Youk EG. Endoscopic treatment of large colorectal tumors: comparison of endoscopic mucosal resection, endoscopic mucosal resection-precutting, and endoscopic submucosal dissection. Surg Endosc. 2012;26(8):2220 30.

53. Wang J, Zhang XH, Ge J, Yang CM, Liu JY, Zhao SL. Endoscopic submucosal dissection vs endoscopic mucosal resection for colorectal tumors: a meta-analysis. World J Gastroenterol. 2014;20(25):8282–7.

54. Moss A, Williams SJ, Hourigan LF, Brown G, Tam W, Singh R, et al. Long-term adenoma recurrence following wide-field endoscopic mucosal resection (WF-EMR) for advanced colonic mucosal neoplasia is infrequent: results and risk factors in 1000 cases from the Australian colonic EMR (ACE) study. Gut. 2015;64(1):57–65.

55. Repici A, Hassan C, De Pessoa DP, Pagano N, Arezzo A, Zullo A, et al. Efficacy and safety of endoscopic submucosal dissection for colorectal neoplasia: a systematic review. Endoscopy. 2012;44(2):137–50.

56. Cipolletta L, Rotondano G, Bianco MA, Buffoli F, Gizzi G, Tessari F, et al. Endoscopic resection for superficial colorectal neoplasia in Italy: a prospective multicentre study. Dig Liver Dis. 2014;46(2):146–51.

57. Kudo S, Lambert R, Allen JI, Fujii H, Fujii T, Kashida H, et al. Nonpolypoid neoplastic lesions of the colorectal mucosa. Gastrointest Endosc. 2008;68(4 Suppl):S3–47.

58. Lambert R, Kudo SE, Vieth M, Allen JI, Fujii H, Fujii T, et al. Pragmatic classification of superficial neoplastic colorectal lesions. Gastrointest Endosc. 2009;70(6):1182–99.

59. Watanabe T, Itabashi M, Shimada Y, Tanaka S, Ito Y, Ajioka Y, et al. Japanese Society for Cancer of the colon and Rectum (JSCCR) guidelines 2010 for the treatment of colorectal cancer. Int J Clin Oncol. 2012;17(1):1–29.

Colonoscopic Polypectomy: Current Techniques and Controversies

4

Fabio Monica and Giulia Maria Pecoraro

4.1 Introduction

Colonoscopic polypectomy is a well-recognized method for the prevention of colorectal cancer (CRC), reducing its incidence [1] and mortality [2].

The first polypectomy was performed in 1969 by Dr. Hiromi Shinya, a general surgeon working at Beth Israel Hospital in New York, using an electrosurgical polypectomy snare that he designed. The results were published a few years later in the *New England Journal of Medicine* and this article became known as one of the twentieth century's landmark articles in the field [3].

Despite their proven effectiveness, polyp resection techniques are based on expert opinion and uncontrolled observational studies and are limited by a lack of evidence [4–6]. Moreover, there is no standardized polypectomy method, so that most endoscopists perform polypectomy as they have learned during their endoscopic training or advanced fellowship. In 2004 a survey conducted among American gastroenterologists showed substantial variation in polypectomy practices even for lesions less than 10 mm [7–9]. Proper removal of polyps needs not only the skills of an experienced endoscopist but also a complete knowledge of the characteristics of endoscopic instruments and accessories, according to their suitability for the morphology and size of the colorectal polyp, in order to avoid complications and to reduce the occurrence of incomplete polypectomy, which is one of the major causes of interval colon cancer [10, 11].

In the CRC screening era, detection and resection of all polypoid lesions are the main goals of quality colonoscopy, and submitting all resected polyps to histological examination is still the standard of care [12, 13].

F. Monica (✉) • G.M. Pecoraro
Division of Gastroenterology and Digestive Endoscopy, Azienda Sanitaria Universitaria Integrata di Trieste, Academic Hospital Cattinara, Trieste, Italy
e-mail: monifabio@gmail.com

© Springer International Publishing AG 2018
A. Facciorusso, N. Muscatiello (eds.), *Colon Polypectomy*,
https://doi.org/10.1007/978-3-319-59457-6_4

Before performing a polypectomy it is necessary to determine whether the patient is receiving anticoagulant/antiplatelet therapy to assess for bleeding risk, as shown in the American Society for Gastrointestinal Endoscopy guidelines (2016) [14]. (For this topic please refer to Chap. 9.)

4.2 Polypectomy Techniques

A successful polypectomy has to be effective in achieving complete resection, efficient in the retrieval of all lesions, and safe in minimizing the risk of complications such as perforation or bleeding. Furthermore, the resection must provide an accurate histological diagnosis, with evaluation of the margins and investigation for possible neoplastic invasion of the underlying layers.

Several techniques are used to remove polyps; they are classified according to the accessories used, with or without the use of electrosurgery. The choice of technique depends on the morphology, size, and location of the polyps and the experience of the endoscopist [15, 16].

Classification of colorectal polyps is critical to facilitate a standardized approach to therapy [13, 17, 18]. At present, superficial neoplastic lesions of the gastrointestinal tract are stratified into three categories according to the Paris endoscopic classification: protruded (type 0-I), superficial (type 0–II), and excavated (type 0–III). Protruded lesions are subdivided into pedunculated (0-Ip), if the polyps have a head connected with a stalk; sessile (0-Is), if the polyps are broad-based without a connecting stalk; and semipedunculated (0-Isp) if the polyps have short stalk [19–21]. Based on size it is possible to identify three types of polyps: diminutive, ≤ 5 mm; intermediate, between 6 and 9 mm; and large, >10 mm.

The endoscopic techniques for polypectomy are:

1. Cold forceps biopsy (CFB)
2. Hot forceps biopsy (HFB)
3. Snare excision: cold snare polypectomy (CSP) and hot snare polypectomy (with monopolar cautery [HSP])
4. Simple fulguration with argon plasma coagulation (APC) and advanced techniques such as endoscopic mucosal resection (EMR) and endoscopic submucosal dissection (ESD), which are discussed in the next chapter.

The optimal method for polypectomy is the removal of the polyp in one piece (en-bloc resection), but if the size of the polyp is larger than 2 cm, it may be necessary to remove it in multiple pieces (piecemeal resection).

4.2.1 Cold Forceps Biopsy

The cold forceps technique is easy to use, and has a high retrieval rate and a low complication rate [22]. The distance between cups determines the size of the

Fig. 4.1 Jumbo forceps

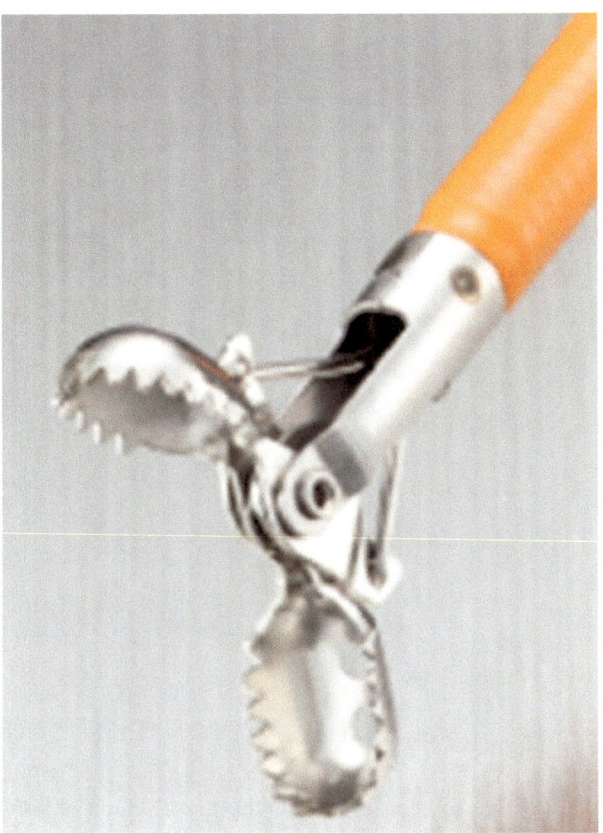

forceps (5–8 mm). The diameter of the forceps cup is about 3 mm. In jumbo forceps the cup size is greater than 3 mm (Fig. 4.1).

The cold forceps technique is used most often for diminutive lesions ($\leq$5 mm) and consists of grasping the polyp and removing it with a firm pull. This allows safe retrieval. Nevertheless, one-bite forceps polypectomy is not always adequate because it may leave residual polyp (also, the exact margins of the polyp may be obscured by blood), so two bites can be done with standard forceps, or, for the complete removal of 4- to 5-mm polyps, jumbo forceps can be used [13, 23, 24]. In two-bite cold forceps polypectomy, the first bite should include a normal mucosal margin to reduce remnant tissue.

A recent prospective study showed that forceps ensured complete resection in 96% of cases for polyps between 1 and 3 mm and in 76% of cases for polyps between 4 and 5 mm [25]. Another study demonstrated that residual adenoma was present in 29% of diminutive polyp sites [26]. Even jumbo forceps seem to be associated with a high rate of residual adenoma [27].

However, another study has shown that complete resection was achieved in 90% of diminutive polyps and 100% of polyps <3 mm in size when performed with chromoendoscopy and washing and post-resection examination [28]. In any case, the endoscopist should always examine the biopsy site to ensure complete removal.

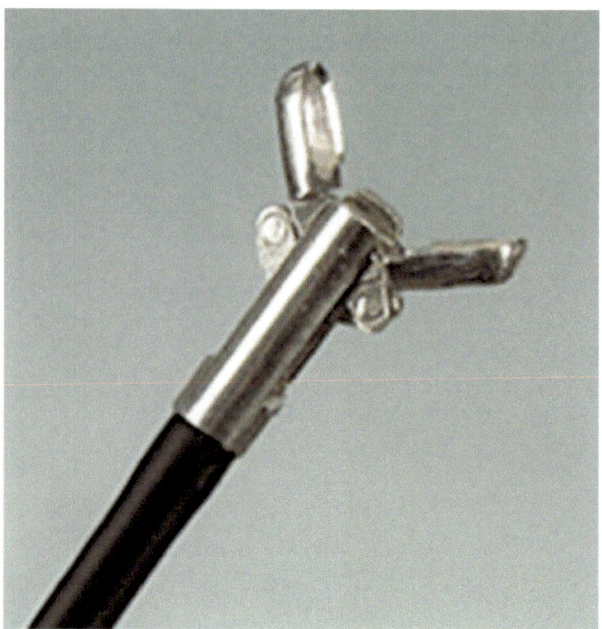

Fig. 4.2 Hot biopsy

4.2.2 Hot Forceps Biopsy

HFB (Fig. 4.2) consists of the thermal ablation of polyps with a coagulation current through an electrosurgical unit, so it is similar to CFB except for its use of electrocautery to remove polyp tissue. When the polyp is grasped in the forceps, electrocautery is applied to destroy the polyp base, while the polyp tissue is preserved inside the forceps as a histological specimen. However, the use of HFB can make histological diagnosis difficult and it has a risk of delayed bleeding or hypercoagulation syndrome [12, 29, 30]. A prospective randomized clinical trial [31] compared the efficacy and safety of CSP and HFB for diminutive colorectal polyps in 287 patients, evaluating endoscopic en-bloc resection and complete histological resection rates (primary outcome), and complication and polyp retrieval rates (secondary outcomes). The authors concluded that CSP is more effective and safer than HFB for diminutive polyps. For these reasons HFB is not recommended as a standard method.

4.2.3 Snare Excision

Snare excision is commonly used for polyps ≥6 mm [7, 32]. Different types of wire loop snares are available, differing according to shape (round, oval, hexagonal, asymmetrical) (Fig. 4.3), according to filament (monofilament or double-stranded) (Fig. 4.4), and according to size (10, 13, 15, 20, 22, 27, and 30 mm) (Fig. 4.5). All of

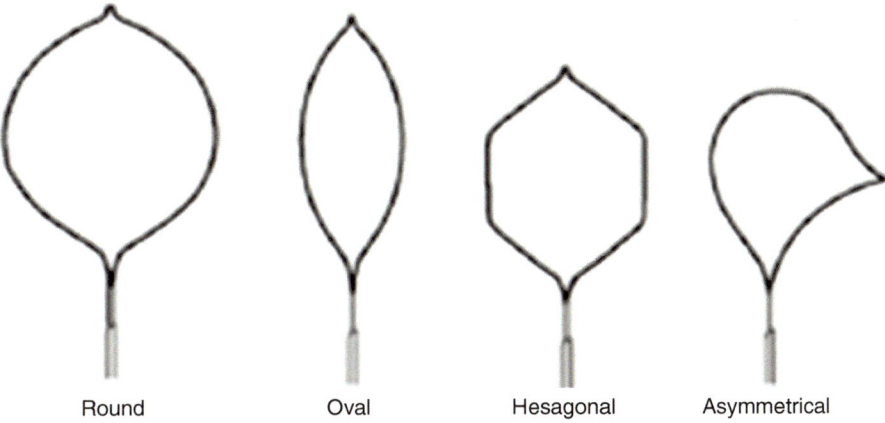

Round   Oval   Hesagonal   Asymmetrical

Fig. 4.3 Various shapes of snares

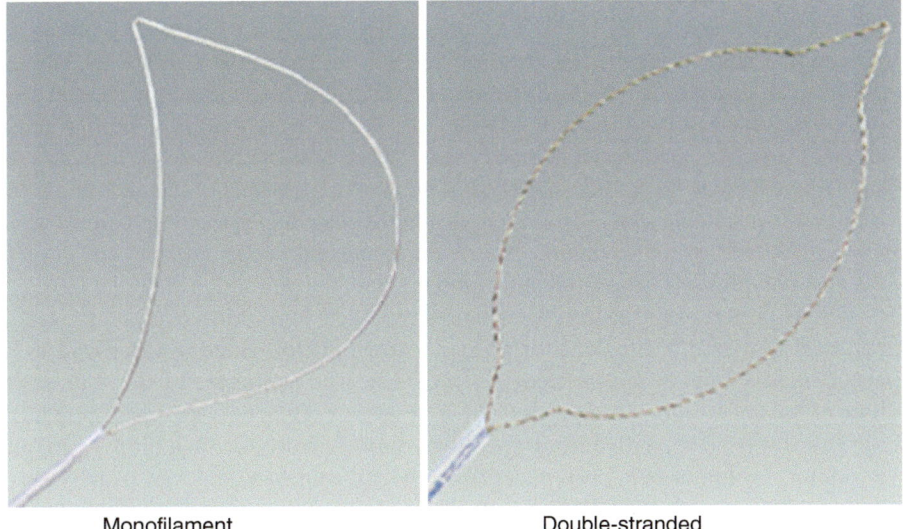

Monofilament   Double-stranded

Fig. 4.4 Various types of filament

these snares can be either soft or stiff. Other specific snare types have also been developed, such as barbed snares (oval snares with spikes or spiral snares) to ensure a firm grasp or prevent slippage of flat or sessile polyps, spiral snares with an incorporated retrieval device, and rotatable snares [33]. The choice of snare is usually made according to the endoscopist's preference as there are no controlled trials demonstrating the superiority of any one device over another.

There are two ways to use the snare: cold snare and standard snare excision with electrocautery.

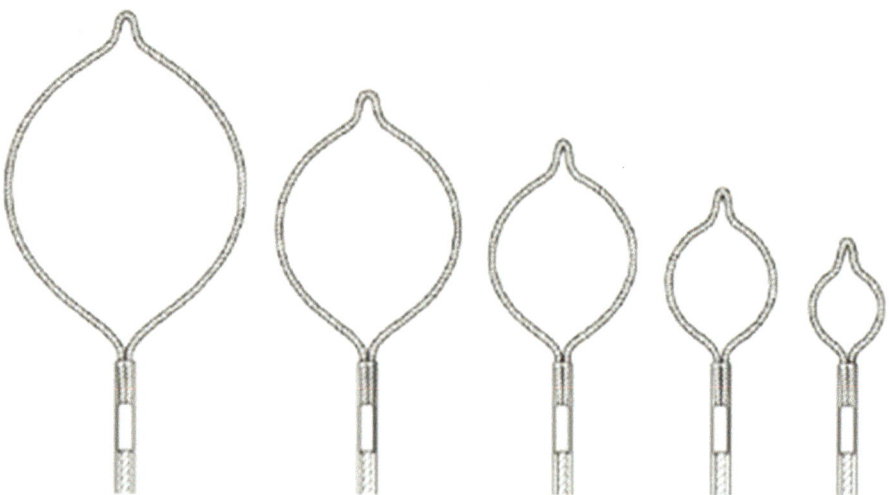

Fig. 4.5 Various sizes of snares

The first method is when the endoscopist decides to cut the polyp with only the mechanical strength of the snare, which is closed in a single, continuous, and controlled movement to guillotine the tissue, also capturing 1–2 mm of normal tissue around the polyp. Suction can help the snare to capture the polyp and surrounding tissue. The polyp can be readily suctioned in the working channel of the endoscope and retrieved in a suitable trap [34]. If there is minimal bleeding, successful hemostasis is always achieved by the technique of positioning the endoscope 'en face' and close to the post-polypectomy base or creating pressure with the power of a water jet [35].

CSP is preferred for lesions less than 10 mm (4–9 mm). Moreover, it also seems better for polyps ≤5 mm, as shown in a recent study, in which it was found to be adequate for complete and safe polyp removal, as well as shortening the withdrawal time of the colonoscopy procedure [36]. CSP allows efficient resection of polyp tissue in a single piece, with a lower rate of incomplete resection than biopsy [26] and it is almost without risk [34], except for insignificant bleeding that usually stops within a few seconds [36]. Repici et al., in an observational study, demonstrated the safety of the cold snare for polyps less than 10 mm, with a low rate of bleeding (1.8%) and no delayed bleeding or perforation [37]. If there is some bleeding, especially in patients taking anticoagulants, it is immediately displayed and can be treated endoscopically.

In view of these findings for CSP, and because of the high rates of incomplete resection with CBF excision, the European Society of Gastrointestinal Endoscopy (ESGE) guidelines now recommend against the use of CBF excision. Only in the case of a polyp sized 1–3 mm where cold snare polypectomy is difficult or not possible, CBF may be used [38].

HSP, i.e., standard snare excision with monopolar cautery, is the most widely used technique for polyps of 10–19 mm and it has been used for about 40 years [39, 40].

Despite this long history, the application of electrocautery in snare polypectomy has not yet been standardized because of the lack of large controlled trials (see Sect. 2.3.4).

4.2.3.1 Saline Lift Technique

To make HSP effective and safe it may be aided by the saline lift technique, which prepares the polyps for resection. With a suitable needle, saline solution (or other agents that are retained for longer periods) can be injected into the submucosa under the polyp, raising the lesion from the underlying muscularis propria.

This has the dual purpose of increasing the distance between the polyp and the submucosa, ensuring complete removal of the polyp and reducing the risk of complications [41]. This method potentially decreases the risk of perforation because the electric current will be conducted within a greater tissue space. Further more, most endoscopists use dilute epinephrine (1:10,000 or 1:20,000) to reduce the risk of bleeding, taking advantage of its vasoconstrictor properties.

Unfortunately, saline solution is rapidly absorbed, so alternative agents have been studied, including hyaluronic acid [42], dextrose solution [43], succinylated gelatin [44], hydroxyethyl starch [45], and recently polidocanol [46]; these are used with or without epinephrine. (For this topic please refer to Chap. 7).

4.2.3.2 Steps for Performing Polypectomy

When performing endoscopic polypectomy with a snare, some steps should be kept in mind.

Correct Position

The polyp should always be placed in the 5- to 7 o'clock position.

Identification of the polyp margins: High-definition/resolution endoscopes with electronic chromoendoscopy (Narrow Banding Imaging (NBI), Olympus Corporation, Tokyo, Japan; Fuji Intelligent Chromo Endoscopy (FICE), Fujifilm Corporation, Tokyo, Japan; Blue Light Imaging (BLI), Fujifilm Corporation, Tokyo, Japan; iSCAN, Pentax Corporation, Tokyo, Japan) help to provide clear visualization of the polyp margins. Adding biologically inert blue dye (methylene blue or indigo carmine) to the saline used to lift the polyp helps in defining the borders of a flat/sessile lesion.

Infiltration of the submucosa (*optional if HSP is used*): This must always be started in the proximal part (anatomically) of the polyp base, so that the polyp will rise from the side of the vision and will not tip over.

Ensnaring (Trapping)

The tip of the snare should be placed proximal to the fold; the nurse then opens the snare slowly, surrounding the polyp, and then the snare is slowly closed while the catheter tip is simultaneously advanced at the base of the polyp, keeping the tip in position. This allows the trapping of the entire polyp base and prevents the snare from slipping back over the head of the polyp when it is closed. Gentle suction during snare closure facilitates the entrapment of a completely flat lesion, but it must be done carefully to avoid clasping too much tissue or a colonic fold.

Resection

The snare is completely closed to cut the polyp with electrocautery.

When electrocautery is used the endoscopist should minimize the duration of energy delivery to limit damage to the colonic wall. Every part ensnared should be lifted away from the wall: this can be done by tenting the polyp toward the center of the lumen just before the application of the current, to prevent deep perforation. Furthermore, we must be careful that the tip of the snare does not inadvertently touch the wall behind the polyp, because if this happens thermal injury with delayed perforation may occur.

Retrieval

If the pieces are relatively small they can be suctioned through the suction channel [34]; otherwise, an endoscopic net, wire basket, or forceps can be used for the retrieval of a large resected polyp or tissue that will not pass through the channel, especially if the polyp is located in the right colon.

The optimal method of removal for large polyps (>1 cm) varies with the type of polyp, so it is important to identify large pedunculated or sessile polyps and flat lesions.

4.2.3.3 Polypectomy for Different Types of Polyps

Most pedunculated polyps develop large feeding blood vessels in the stalk [47], and the size of these vessels may be greater than the size of the polyp and its stalk.

When removing pedunculated polyps, applying energy early and closing the snare slowly will help to avoid complications such as bleeding. The electrocautery snare should be placed around the stalk at approximately one-half to one-third of the distance between the polyp head and the colon wall, allowing sufficient resection margin in case there is malignancy and leaving a visible residual stump of the stalk after resection that can be grasped in the event of bleeding.

To prevent bleeding, it is useful to place a nylon loop (Endoloop, Olympus Corporation, Tokyo, japan) [48] around the stalk below the resection point (even if the presence of this loop may make the procedure challenging) or to place clips across the polyp stalk.

Bleeding rates increase when the stalk is >5 mm [47]. However, the size threshold for the prophylactic application of mechanical measures to prevent bleeding is not known. The ESGE guidelines recommended that, for a pedunculated polyp with a head ≥20 mm or a stalk ≥10 mm in diameter, it is useful to pretreat the stalk with these mechanical measures for hemostasis and/or to use an injection of dilute epinephrine [38].

No difference in efficacy between clips and a nylon loop for the prophylaxis of bleeding is currently known [49].

Large sessile polyps are difficult to remove and polyps greater than 2 cm are usually removed in a piecemeal manner or by using advanced techniques.

In order to perform the polypectomy in a correct and safe way, the endoscopist must know and apply the electrical current that is the most suitable for the type and size of polyp to be removed.

Table 4.1 Endoscopic techniques according to the feature of polyps

Size and type of polyp	Technique	Instrument	Other accessories
3–4 mm	Cold forceps (one-bite) Hot forceps (not recommended)	Forceps	–
5–6 mm	Cold forceps (two-bite)	Forceps or jumbo forceps	–
7–9 mm	Cold snare	Mini oval snare, barbed snare	–
	Hot snare		Injection needle (optional)
Large pedunculated	Hot snare	Braided-soft	Injection needle, Endoloop, clip
Large sessile	Hot snare	Braided-stiff	Injection needle
Flat lesion	Hot snare	Monofilament	Injection needle

Traditionally, snare polypectomy is performed using a blended, coagulation, or pure cutting electrical current. Table 4.1 summarizes the endoscopic techniques according to the feature of polyps.

4.2.3.4 Electrosurgery Unit (ESU)

The basic principle of the ESU is that heat can be produced without a neuromuscular response when a high-frequency alternating current between 300 kHz and 3 mHz (radiofrequency) passes through tissue. The ESU is a commonly used endoscopic tool for cutting or coagulating tissue. Depending on the wave form chosen, energy applied at the cellular level produces heat because of tissue resistance, resulting in the bursting of cell membranes, with tissue disruption or coagulation being caused by a less intense electrical current, which can desiccate and shrink cells without bursting the cell membrane, while providing hemostasis [12, 13].

Monopolar devices transmit current from an electrode in the instrument tip through the patient's body to a plate (usually placed on the leg or thigh) to complete the circuit; bipolar devices have both active and return electrodes in the instrument tip, thereby foregoing the need for a grounding plate.

Various types of ESU have been developed, depending on the current used; for example, pure coagulation current and pure cutting current. However, these methods involve complications, because coagulation current may be associated with perforation, owing to the deep tissue penetration of heat, whereas the use of cutting current has a risk of immediate post-polypectomy bleeding because the tissues are cut before vessels are coagulated. Therefore, engineers have developed a blended current that modulates the frequency of the electrical current (duty cycle) and adjusts the peak voltage. The result is that the current exerts a cutting effect on the tissue with a coagulating effect at the resected margin [39]. Specific tools have been developed to facilitate controlled tissue cutting during various applications, alternating cutting and coagulation currents.

The blended current can be provided by a conventional electrosurgical generator or by using a generator with a microprocessor that automatically controls currents, fractionates cutting and coagulating phases, and adjusts output based on tissue impedance, with the result being the restriction of deep tissue injury.

Improvements in technology have seen the introduction of more sophisticated electrosurgical generators in which the ENDO CUT mode (Erbe, Elektromedizin GmbH, Tubingen, Germany) has been widely used because of its better results for polypectomy, as it rapidly modifies the current in response to changes in the tissue impedance. Alternating cutting and coagulation cycles allow controlled cutting to be performed with sufficient hemostasis during the entire cutting process, with minimal depth and spread of thermal injury. For more effective cutting or deeper coagulation, the endoscopist can adjust different parameters: the coagulation power, the cut duration, and the interval between the previous and next cut [14].

Some studies have shown that, overall, the ENDO CUT is better than a conventional electrosurgical generator in terms of the quality of the polypectomy specimens and the less extensive tissue damage [50].

However, electrosurgery is responsible for almost all the complications associated with polypectomy [51] and there are no uniform or standard guidelines for electrosurgical settings during polypectomy.

4.2.3.5 New Methods

Recently "underwater" polypectomy has been used during water-aided colonoscopy. This technique for the removal of flat colorectal lesions was described for the first time by Dr. Kenneth Binmoeller and colleagues, in 2012 [52].

The bowel lumen is filled with water rather than air, and a submucosal injection of the lesion is not required. This technique increases the complete resection rate and reduces possible complications: bleeding, transmural burns, and perforation. Both cold and hot snares can be used safely because water does not affect the conductivity of the tissue during polypectomy. However, further studies are needed to validate the technique.

In recent years the use of carbon dioxide insufflation during polypectomy has developed too. This seems to reduce patient discomfort during and after the procedure because CO_2 is absorbed faster than air [53, 54].

4.2.4   Argon Plasma Coagulation

Argon plasma coagulation should be used for the electrocautery of islets of adenomatous tissue between resected pieces or polypectomy margins, but its efficacy is unclear because this method is associated with polyp recurrence [20, 55]. This technology uses a non-flammable and inexpensive gas: ionized argon (plasma). A jet of ionized argon is emitted by 6000-volt peak energy. Thermal energy is conducted by argon and delivered into the tissue with a depth of penetration of roughly 2–3 mm, producing denatured proteins, with the net effect being tissue destruction and coagulation. The tip of the probe must be oriented less than 1 cm from the target lesion and it is important not to fire too close to the mucosa, because the coagulation effect is similar to that of monopolar electrocautery rather than the effect achieved via ionizing plasma, which causes deeper injury of the tissue.

4.3   Controversies

4.3.1   Incomplete Resection

There are two important issues with polypectomy: incomplete resection and non-retrieval of the polyp. Surveillance intervals are based on complete removal of all adenomas, while in cases of incomplete polypectomy, residual neoplastic tissue can progress to malignancy. It has been estimated that up to 27% of interval cancers may occur owing to incomplete endoscopic resection [10, 56].

The CARE study [57] showed that residual adenoma was common after HSP, and rates of incomplete resection varied according to the type and size of the polyps: there were high rates (over 10%) for non-pedunculated neoplastic polyps, and the rates of incomplete resection were 6.8% for polyps 6–9 mm, 17.8% for polyps 10–20 mm, and 31.0% for sessile serrated polyps. In another study, 17.6% of patients with large sessile polyps had residual adenomatous tissue when reexamined [58].

Of note, the CARE study [57] concluded that the rates of incomplete resection varied significantly among endoscopists (6.5–22.7%), suggesting that the individual operator factor and appropriate training are the most important factors for correct and successful polypectomy [59, 60].

A survey of 189 gastroenterologists showed there was no agreement on a technique for the removal of 4- to 6-mm polyps. For polyps 1–3 mm in size, forceps techniques (cold or hot) were more frequently used and for polyps 7–9 mm in size electrosurgical snare resection was predominant, whereas for polyps measuring 4–6 mm, 19% of the respondents reported using cold biopsy forceps, 21% hot biopsy forceps, 59% a hot snare, and 15% a cold snare. Thus, for polyps 4–6 mm in size no one polypectomy method was used significantly more than any other method [7].

Prospective randomized comparisons are required to assess the efficacy and safety of cold-snare polypectomy versus cold biopsy in lesions 4–6 mm and of cold forceps versus HSP, particularly in lesions 6–9 mm.

4.3.2   Non-retrieval of Polyps

Another issue is the non-retrieval of polyps; this prevents pathological evaluation of the resected polyp, which is one of the criteria for surveillance intervals. Generally, the percentage of polyps lost after resection ranges from 2.1 to 19% [61, 62]. The biopsy techniques provide high polyp retrieval rates (95–100%) [25, 61]. On the other hand, in one retrospective study, about 13% of smaller polyps (1–5 mm) and 19% of polyps overall removed by cold-snare, were not retrieved [63].

The optimal retrieval strategy has not been defined, although some factors were independently associated with non-retrieval: previous colorectal surgery, resection by cold snare, location in the right colon, inadequate bowel preparation, and a polyp size up to 5 mm [63, 64]. In a retrospective study, 4383 removed polyps were analyzed in terms of the polyp features (number, size, and location), removal technique, bowel preparation, and quality of the colonoscopy (duration of examination, insertion, and withdrawal). Multivariate analysis showed that the independent factors for non-retrieval of polyps were small size and cold-snare removal. Other factors correlated with non-retrieval were sessile polyps and location in the proximal colon. In this study the number of polyps per patient, quality of bowel preparation, and duration of the procedure were also correlated with the retrieval rate [63].

The American Society for Gastrointestinal Endoscopy [65] has formulated new paradigms for the colonoscopic management of diminutive (5 mm in size) colorectal polyps that may reduce costs and improve patient safety compared with the current paradigm. The first paradigm ("resect and discard") refers to polyps that are removed and discarded so that the endoscopic assessment of histology is done to establish future surveillance; the second paradigm proposes to leave in situ all diminutive polyps in the rectosigmoid colon when the endoscopist has established a hyperplastic pattern. There are some criticisms in regard to adopting this strategy and it is still under investigation.

Finally, providing education and feedback to endoscopists will improve polyp retrieval rates, especially for clinically relevant, right-sided polyps [66].

4.4 Polyps that are difficult to approach

When we are faced with a polyp that is difficult to approach owing to its location in a tight turn or behind a colonic fold, we can employ some strategies, such as locking the dials on the endoscope or asking an assistant to maintain the scope position (for polyps in tight bends), performing retroflexion of the scope tip (only in the right colon), or using a side-viewing duodenoscope [67, 68] or cap-assisted colonoscope for polyps behind folds. However, no standardized guideline exists for the removal of such polyps, and the choice of method depends on the experience and preference of the operator.

Sometimes polypectomy can be difficult in the presence of submucosal fibrosis caused by previous attempts at resection or even injudicious biopsies. In such cases the submucosal injection of saline solution does not ensure the lifting of the polyp, because the mucosa and submucosa adhere to the underlying muscularis propria, and incomplete removal occurs with snare polypectomy [69]. Thus, for polyps that are difficult to approach, it is mandatory to do a complete resection in one session and never perform biopsies on the polyps. If you are not able to do this, it is preferable to refer the patient to a tertiary center.

4.5 Tattooing

After polypectomy it is necessary to assess whether there is an opportunity to make a tattoo of the lesion site, especially when the polyp was large, if we are not sure that removal was complete, or if other sessions will be needed to remove it, and if there are indicators suspicious of malignancy. The tattooing procedure allows simple and accurate identification of the polypectomy site. However, if the lesion is located in the rectum, in the cecum, or near the ileocecal valve, the site should not be tattooed [38].

Although tattooing is not done routinely at the time of the initial procedure, some endoscopists prefer to tattoo all large polypectomy sites at the time of the initial procedure because of the inherent risk of harboring malignancies [70].

Tattooing consists of the injection of a permanent staining agent into the gut wall to create a mark that will identify the site from either inside or outside the lumen; it is typically done with at least two submucosal injections of dye on contralateral sides of the bowel near the lesion. The tattooing should be done a few centimeters distal to the lesion or at three or four sites circumferentially to avoid the risk of tumor seeding [71].

The needle should ideally enter the mucosa at an oblique angle to permit injection into the submucosa rather than penetrating the colon wall, which can result in inflammation and diffuse staining of the peritoneum, thereby obscuring the surgeon's view during operation [72]. If a submucosal bleb is not immediately developed during the injection, the needle should be pulled back slightly while dye continues to be injected until a bleb is seen [73].

More recently some endoscopists have performed a double injection, with a saline injection into the submucosa to form a bleb, followed by an injection of dye using a second syringe. It seems that this technique can improve the efficacy of tattooing and prevent inflammatory complications [74, 75].

Many types of dye are available for tattooing (including methylene blue, indigo carmine, toluidine blue, and hematoxylin), but only two persist for more than 24 h: indocyanine green and India ink [76].

The latter is widely adopted, but some complications related to India ink solution injection have been described. In addition to intraperitoneal spillage (reported in up to 14% of cases, but rarely with any clinical significance), there have been reports of perforation leading to peritonitis [77], abscess formation [78], fat necrosis [79], phlegmonous gastritis [80], inflammatory pseudotumour [81], accidental marking of the small bowel or inadvertent staining of the entire sigmoid colon [82], and abscess in the rectus muscle [83]. Also, India ink is not a sterile solution.

More recently a dilute suspension of pure carbon particles (SPOT® Gi Supply, Camp Hill, PA USA) has been developed as a sterile and biocompatible suspension. This is the only dye approved by the Food and Drug Administration of the United States and it is efficient and safe. However, cases of peritonitis and submucosal fibrosis have been reported with this suspension [84].

References

1. Winawer SJ, Zauber AG, Ho MN, O'Brien MJ, Gottlieb LS, Sternberg SS, Waye JD, Schapiro M, Bond JH, Panish JF, et al. Prevention of colorectal cancer by colonoscopic polypectomy. The National Polyp Study Workgroup. N Engl J Med. 1993;329(27):1977–81.
2. Zauber AG, Winawer SJ, O'Brien MJ, Lansdorp-Vogelaar I, van Ballegooijen M, Hankey BF, Shi W, Bond JH, Schapiro M, Panish JF, Stewart ET, Waye JD. Colonoscopic polypectomy and long-term prevention of colorectal-cancer deaths. N Engl J Med. 2012;366(8):687–96.

3. Wolff WI, Shinya H. Polypectomy via the fiberoptic colonoscope. Removal of neoplasms beyond reach of the sigmoidoscope. N Engl J Med. 1973;288(7):329–32.
4. Rex DK. Have we defined best colonoscopic polypectomy practice in the United States? Clin Gastroenterol Hepatol. 2007;5:674–7.
5. Hewett DG, Rex DK. Colonoscopy and diminutive polyps: hot or cold biopsy or snare? Do I send to pathology? Clin Gastroenterol Hepatol. 2011;9:102–5.
6. Pattullo V, Bourke MJ, Tran KL, et al. The suction pseudopolyp technique: a novel method for the removal of small flat nonpolypoid lesions of the colon and rectum. Endoscopy. 2009;41:1032.
7. Singh N, Harrison M, Rex DK. A survey of colonoscopic polypectomy practices among clinical gastroenterologists. Gastrointest Endosc. 2004;99:414–8.
8. Gupta S, Anderson J, Bhandari P, et al. Development and validation of a novel method for assessing competency in polypectomy: direct observation of polypectomy skills. Gastrointest Endosc. 2011;73:1232–9.
9. Gupta S, Bassett P, Man R, et al. Validation of a novel method for assessing competency in polypectomy. Gastrointest Endosc. 2012;75:568–75.
10. Pabby A, Schoen RE, Weissfeld JL, Burt R, Kikendall JW, Lance P, Shike M, Lanza E, Schatzkin A. Analysis of colorectal cancer occurrence during surveillance colonoscopy in the dietary polyp prevention trial. Gastrointest Endosc. 2005;61(3):385–91.
11. Farrar WD, Sawhney MS, Nelson DB, Lederle FA, Bond JH. Colorectal cancers found after a complete colonoscopy. Clin Gastroenterol Hepatol. 2006;4(10):1259–64.
12. Park HJ. Endoscopic instruments and electrosurgical unit for colonoscopic polypectomy. Clin Endosc. 2016;49:350–4.
13. Kedia P, Waye JD. Colon polypectomy: a review of routine and advanced techniques. J Clin Gastroenterol. 2013;47(8):657–65.
14. Carter D, Beer-Gabel M, Eliakim R, Novis B, Avidan B, Bardan E. Management of antithrombotic agents for colonoscopic polypectomies in Israeli gastroenterologists relative to published guidelines. Clin Res Hepatol Gastroenterol. 2013;37(5):514–8.
15. Weinberg DS. Large adenoma recurrence after polypectomy. Gastrointest Endosc. 2009;70:350–2.
16. Bae GH, Jung JT, Kwon JG, et al. Risk factors of delayed bleeding after colonoscopic polypectomy: case-control study. Korean J Gastroenterol. 2012;59:423–7.
17. Bourke M. Current status of colonic endoscopic mucosal resection in the west and the interface with endoscopic submucosal dissection. Dig Endosc. 2009;21(Suppl 1):S22–7.
18. Lambert R, Kudo SE, Vieth M, et al. Pragmatic classification of superficial colorectal neoplastic lesions. Gastrointest Endosc. 2009;70:1182–99.
19. Participants in the Paris Workshop. The Paris endoscopic classification of superficial neoplastic lesions: esophagus, stomach, and colon. Gastrointest Endosc. 2003;58(Suppl 6):S3–43.
20. Endoscopic Classification Review Group. Update on the Paris classification of superficial neoplastic lesions in the digestive tract. Endoscopy. 2005;37(6):570–8.
21. Macrae FA. Approach to the patient with colonic polyps. UpToDate. 2017.
22. Rex DK. Preventing colorectal cancer and cancer mortality with colonoscopy: what we know and what we don't know. Endoscopy. 2010;42:320–3.
23. Draganov PV, Chang MN, Alkhasawneh A, et al. Randomized, controlled trial of standard, large-capacity versus jumbo biopsy forceps for polypectomy of small, sessile, colorectal polyps. Gastrointest Endosc. 2012;75:118–26.
24. Uraoka T, Matsuda T, Sano Y, et al. Polypectomy using jumbo biopsy forceps for small colorectal polyps: a multicenter prospective trial. Gastrointest Endosc. 2013;77:AB564.
25. Lee CK, Shim JJ, Jang JY. Cold snare polypectomy vs. cold forceps polypectomy using double-biopsy technique for removal of diminutive colorectal polyps: a prospective randomized study. Am J Gastroenterol. 2013;108:1593–600.
26. Woods A, Sanowski RA, Wadas DD, et al. Eradication of diminutive polyps: a prospective evaluation of bipolar coagulation versus conventional biopsy removal. Gastrointest Endosc. 1989;35:536–40.

27. Draganov PV, Chang MN, Lieb J, et al. Randomized controlled trial of two types of biopsy forceps for polypectomy of small sessile colorectal polyps. Gastrointest Endosc. 2010;71:AB194.
28. Jung YS, Park JH, Kim HJ, et al. Complete biopsy resection of diminutive polyps. Endoscopy. 2013;45:1024–9.
29. Monkemuller KE, Fry LC, Jones BH, Wells C, Mikolaenko I, Eloubeidi M. Histological quality of polyps resected using the cold versus hot biopsy technique. Endoscopy. 2004;36:432–6.
30. Lee SH, Shin SJ, Park DI, et al. Korean guideline for colonoscopic polypectomy. Clin Endosc. 2012;45:11–24.
31. Komeda Y, Kashida H, Sakurai T, Tribonias G, Okamoto K, Kono M, Yamada M, Adachi T, Mine H, Nagai T, Asakuma Y, Hagiwara S, Matsui S, Watanabe T, Kitano M, Chikugo T, Chiba Y, Kudo M. Removal of diminutive colorectal polyps: a prospective randomized clinical trial between cold snare polypectomy and hot forceps biopsy. World J Gastroenterol. 2017;23(2):328–35.
32. Hewett DG. Colonoscopic polypectomy: current techniques and controversies. Gastroenterol Clin N Am. 2013;42:443–58.
33. Yamano H, Matsushita H, Yamanaka K, et al. A study of physical efficacy of different snares for endoscopic mucosal resection. Dig Endosc. 2004;16(Suppl 1):S85–8.
34. Deenadayalu VP, Rex DK. Colon polyp retrieval after cold snaring. Gastrointest Endosc. 2005;62:253–6.
35. Uraoka T, Ramberan H, Matsuda T, Fujii T, Yahagi N. Cold polypectomy techniques for diminutive polyps in the colorectum. Dig Endosc. 2014;26(Suppl. 2):98–103.
36. Paspatis GA, Tribonias G, Konstantinidis K, et al. A prospective randomized comparison of cold vs hot snare polypectomy in the occurrence of postpolypectomy bleeding in small colonic polyps. Colorectal Dis. 2011;13:e345–8.
37. Repici A, Hassan C, Vitetta E, et al. Safety of cold polypectomy for <10 mm polyps at colonoscopy: a prospective multicenter study. Endoscopy. 2012;44:27–31.
38. Ferlitsch M, Moss A, Hassan C, Bhandari P, Dumonceau JM, Paspatis G, Jover R, Langner C, Bronzwaer M, Nalankilli K, Fockens P, Hazzan R, Gralnek IM, Gschwantler M, Waldmann E, Jeschek P, Penz D, Heresbach D, Moons L, Lemmers A, Paraskeva K, Pohl J, Ponchon T, Regula J, Repici A, Rutter MD, Burgess NG, Bourke MJ. Colorectal polypectomy and endoscopic mucosal resection (EMR): European Society Of Gastrointestinal Endoscopy (ESGE) clinical guideline. Endoscopy. 2017;49(3):270–97.
39. Morris ML, Tucker RD, Baron TH, et al. Electrosurgery in gastrointestinal endoscopy: principles to practice. Am J Gastroenterol. 2009;104:1563–74.
40. Van Gossum A, Cozzoli A, Adler M, et al. Colonoscopic snare polypectomy: analysis of 1485 resections comparing two types of current. Gastrointest Endosc. 1992;38:472–5.
41. Seitz U, Bohnacker S, Binmoeller KF. Endoscopic removal of large colon polyps. UpToDate. 2017.
42. Friedland S, Kothari S, Chen A, et al. Endoscopic mucosal resection with an over the counter hyaluronate preparation. Gastrointest Endosc. 2012;75:1040.
43. Katsinelos P, Kountouras J, Paroutoglou G, et al. A comparative study of 50% dextrose and normal saline solution on their ability to create submucosal fluid cushions for endoscopic resection of sessile rectosigmoid polyps. Gastrointest Endosc. 2008;68:692.
44. Moss A, Bourke MJ, Metz AJ. A randomized, double-blind trial of succinylated gelatin submucosal injection for endoscopic resection of large sessile polyps of the colon. Am J Gastroenterol. 2010;105:2375.
45. Fasoulas K, Lazaraki G, Chatzimavroudis G, et al. Endoscopic mucosal resection of giant laterally spreading tumors with submucosal injection of hydroxyethyl starch: comparative study with normal saline solution. Surg Laparosc Endosc Percutan Tech. 2012;22:272.
46. Muscatiello N, Facciorusso A. Use of polidocanol in colon polypectomy. Gastrointest Endosc. 2016;83(1):271.
47. Dobrowolski S, Dobosz M, Babicki A, et al. Blood supply of colorectal polyps correlates with risk of bleeding after colonoscopic polypectomy. Gastrointest Endosc. 2006;63:1004–9.
48. Iishi H, Tatsuta M, Narahara H, Iseki K, Sakai N. Endoscopic resection of large pedunculated colorectal polyps using a detachable snare. Gastrointest Endosc. 1996 Nov;44(5):594–7.

49. Ji J-S, Lee S-W, Kim TH, et al. Comparison of prophylactic clip and endoloop application for the prevention of postpolypectomy bleeding in pedunculated colonic polyps: a prospective, randomized, multicenter study. Endoscopy. 2014;46:598–604.
50. Fry LC, Lazenby AJ, Mikolaenko I, Barranco B, Rickes S, Mönkemüller K. Diagnostic quality of polyps resected by snare polypectomy: does the type of electrosurgical current used matter? Am J Gastroenterol. 2006;101(9):2123–7. Epub 2006 Jul 18
51. Ko CW, Dominitz JA. Complications of colonoscopy: magnitude and management. Gastrointest Endosc Clin N Am. 2010;20:659–71.
52. Binmoeller KF, Weilert F, Shah J, Bhat Y, Kane S. "Underwater" EMR without submucosal injection for large sessile colorectal polyps (with video). Gastrointest Endosc. 2012;75(5):1086–91.
53. Wu J, Hu B. The role of carbon dioxide insufflation in colonoscopy: a systematic review and meta-analysis. Endoscopy. 2012;44:128–36.
54. Hsu WF, Hu WH, Chen YN, et al. Carbon dioxide insufflation can significantly reduce toilet use after colonoscopy: a double-blind randomized controlled trial. Endoscopy. 2014;46:190–5.
55. Buchner AM, Guarner-Argente C, Ginsberg GG. Outcomes of EMR of defiant colorectal lesions directed to an endoscopy referral center. Gastrointest Endosc. 2012;76:255–63.
56. Leung K, Pinsky P, Laiyemo AO, et al. Ongoing colorectal cancer risk despite surveillance colonoscopy: the polyp prevention trial continued follow-up study. Gastrointest Endosc. 2010;71:111–7.
57. Pohl H, Srivastava A, Bensen SP, Anderson P, Rothstein RI, Gordon SR, Levy LC, Toor A, Mackenzie TA, Rosch T, Robertson DJ. Incomplete polyp resection during colonoscopy—results of the complete adenoma resection (CARE) study. Gastroenterology. 2013;144(1):74–80.
58. Robertson DJ, Lieberman DA, Winawer SJ, et al. Interval cancer after total colonoscopy: results from a pooled analysis of eight studies. Gastroenterology. 2008;134:A-111–2.
59. Hewett DG, Kahi CJ, Rex DK. Efficacy and effectiveness of colonoscopy: how do we bridge the gap? Gastrointest Endosc Clin N Am. 2010;20:673–84.
60. Adler A, Wegscheider K, Lieberman D, et al. Factors determining the quality of screening colonoscopy: a prospective study on adenoma detection rates, from 12 134 examinations (Berlin colonoscopy project 3, BECOP-3). Gut. 2013;62:236–41.
61. Tsai FC. Strum WB. Prevalence of advanced adenomas in small and diminutive colon polyps using direct measurement of size. Dig Dis Sci. 2011;56(8):2384–8.
62. Kaminski MF, Regula J, Kraszewska E, Polkowski M, Wojciechowska U, Didkowska J, Zwierko M, Rupinski M, Nowacki MP, Butruk E. Quality indicators for colonoscopy and the risk of interval cancer. N Engl J Med. 2010;362(19):1795–803.
63. Komeda Y, Suzuki N, Sarah M, et al. Factors associated with failed polyp retrieval at screening colonoscopy. Gastrointest Endosc. 2013;77:395–400.
64. Fernandes C, Pinho R, Ribeiro I, Silva J, Ponte A, Carvalho J. Risk factors for polyp retrieval failure in colonoscopy. United European Gastroenterol J. 2015;3(4):387–92. https://doi.org/10.1177/2050640615572041.
65. Rex DK, Kahi C, O'Brien M, Levin TR, Pohl H, Rastogi A, Burgart L, Imperiale T, Ladabaum U, Cohen J, Lieberman DA. The American Society for Gastrointestinal Endoscopy PIVI (preservation and incorporation of valuable endoscopic innovations) on real-time endoscopic assessment of the histology of diminutive colorectal polyps. Gastrointest Endosc. 2011;73(3):419–22.
66. Belderbos TD, van Oijen MG, Moons LM, Siersema PD. The "golden retriever" study: improving polyp retrieval rates by providing education and competitive feedback. Gastrointest Endosc. 2016;83(3):596–601. https://doi.org/10.1016/j.gie.2015.07.018. Epub 2015 Aug 29
67. Misra SP, Dwivedi M. Colonoscopy and colonoscopic polypectomy using side-viewing endoscope: a useful, effective and safe procedure. Dig Dis Sci. 2008;53:1285–8.
68. Frimberger E, von Delius S, Rosch T, et al. Colonoscopy and polypectomy with a side-viewing endoscope. Endoscopy. 2007;39:462–5.

69. Burgess NG, Bahin FF, Bourke MJ. Colonic polypectomy (with videos). Gastrointest Endosc. 2015;81(4):813–35.
70. Zafar A, Mustafa M, Chapman M. Colorectal polyps: when should we tattoo? Surg Endosc. 2012;26(11):3264–6.
71. Kang HJ, Lee BI, Kim BW, Choi H, Cho SH, Choi KY, Chae HS, Han SW, Chung IS, Kim KM. Potential cancer cell inoculation of tattoo site through use of a contaminated needle. Gastrointest Endosc. 2006;63(6):884–6.
72. Fasoli A, Pugliese V, Gatteschi B, et al. Endocytoscopic imaging and tattooing: a caveat. Endoscopy. 2009;41(Suppl 2):E41.
73. Adler DG. Tattooing and other methods for localizing colonic lesions. UptoDate. 2017.
74. Sawaki A, Nakamura T, Suzuki T, Hara K, Kato T, Kato T, Hirai T, Kanemitsu Y, Okubo K, Tanaka K, Moriyama I, Kawai H, Katsurahara M, Matsumoto K, Yamao K. A twostep method for marking polypectomy sites in the colon and rectum. Gastrointest Endosc. 2003;57:735–7.
75. Matsushita M, Takakuwa H, Matsubayashi Y. Effective endoscopic tattooing technique. Gastrointest Endosc. 2004;60:165–6.
76. Hammond DC, Lane FR, Welk RA, Madura MJ, Borreson DK, Passinault WJ. Endoscopic tattooing of the colon. An experimental study. Am Surg. 1989;55(7):457–61.
77. Gianom D, Hollinger A, Wirth HP. Intestinal perforation after preoperative colonic tattooing with India ink. Swiss Surg. 2003;9(6):307–10.
78. Park SI, Genta RS, Romeo DP, Weesner RE. Colonic abscess and focal peritonitis secondary to India ink tattooing of the colon. Gastrointest Endosc. 1991;37(1):68–71.
79. Coman E, Brandt LJ, Brenner S, Frank M, Sablay B, Bennett B. Fat necrosis and inflammatory pseudotumor due to endoscopic tattooing of the colon with India ink. Gastrointest Endosc. 1991;37(1):65–8.
80. Singh S, Arif A, Fox C, Basnyat P. Complication after pre-operative India ink tattooing in a colonic lesion. Dig Surg. 2006;23(5–6):303.
81. Hellmig S, Stüber E, Kiehne K, Fölsch UR. Unusual course of colonic tattooing with India ink. Surg Endosc. 2003;17(3):521.
82. Yano H, Okada K, Monden T. Adhesion ileus caused by tattoo-marking: unusual complication after laparoscopic surgery for early colorectal cancer. Dis Colon Rectum. 2003;46(7):987.
83. Alba LM, Pandya PK, Clarkston WK. Rectus muscle abscess associated with endoscopic tattooing of the colon with India ink. Gastrointest Endosc. 2000;52(4):557–8.
84. Askin MP, Waye JD, Fiedler L, Harpaz N. Tattoo of colonic neoplasms in 113 patients with a new sterile carbon compound. Gastrointest Endosc. 2002;56(3):339–42.

Advanced Endoscopic Resection of Colorectal Lesions

5

Jessica X. Yu, Roy Soetikno, and Tonya Kaltenbach

5.1 Introduction

Advanced endoscopic resection techniques are important to ensure adequate removal of complex or large colorectal polyps. Mounting evidence suggests endoscopic resection as a safer, more cost-effective modality [1–3], compared to surgical resection. Multiple society guidelines now recommend endoscopic resection as the first step for the management of complex benign colon polyps. In this article, we will discuss the assessment and technical aspects of advance resection for the management of complex colorectal polyps.

5.2 Polyp Assessment

Determination of submucosal invasion is critical to assess if endoscopic resection is appropriate. Optical diagnosis with macroscopic and microscopic assessment in conjunction with findings such as non-lifting is key to ensuring complete resection.

J.X. Yu
Division of Gastroenterology and Hepatology, Stanford University School of Medicine, Stanford, CA, USA

R. Soetikno
San Francisco Veterans Affairs Medical Center, San Francisco, CA, USA

T. Kaltenbach (✉)
San Francisco Veterans Affairs Medical Center, San Francisco, CA, USA

University of California, San Francisco, San Francisco, CA, USA
e-mail: endoresection@me.com

© Springer International Publishing AG 2018
A. Facciorusso, N. Muscatiello (eds.), *Colon Polypectomy*,
https://doi.org/10.1007/978-3-319-59457-6_5

61

5.2.1   Macroscopic Appearance

Originally described in 2002, the Paris classification categorizes lesion into superficial and advanced types, with type 0 being superficial neoplasms and type 1–5 reserved for advanced carcinoma [4]. Types 0, or superficial neoplasms, are further subclassified into polypoid and non-polypoid lesions (Fig. 5.1). Types 0–I are pedunculated (0-Ip) or sessile (0-Is) in appearance. Type 0-II lesions may be slightly elevated (0-IIa_, flat (0-IIb) or depressed (0-IIc) [4, 5]. Types 0–III are ulcerated lesions.

Morphologic classification is an important step to facilitate lesion management. The risk of submucosal carcinoma is higher for non-polypoid lesions (Paris type 0-II) compared to polypoid lesions [6, 7]. Flat lesions greater than 10 mm are termed laterally spreading tumors (LST) (Fig. 5.1). Granular LSTs (LST-Gs) have a nodular surface appearance as opposed to non-granular LSTs (LST-NGs), which are smooth. LST-Gs with uniform nodules have a <2% submucosal invasion regardless of size. LST-Gs with nonuniform nodules and LST-NGs have higher risk of submucosal invasion [6]. Depressed lesions greater than 20 mm have been found to have a 87.5% risk of submucosal cancer [8].

5.2.2   Microscopic Diagnosis

Real-time optical diagnosis has been found to be highly accurate and effective for the histologic prediction of small colorectal polyps [9]. The Kudo classification describes pit patterns in five categories, using chromoscopy and magnification [10]. Types I and II are nonneoplastic, whereas types III and IV are adenomatous patterns, and type V is cancerous [8]. Narrowband imaging (NBI) can enhance visual assessment of polyps. The NBI International Colorectal Endoscopic (NICE) classification incorporates tissue color, vascular, and surface pattern to differentiate serrated class lesions from adenomatous. It has also been validated for the prediction of submucosal invasion with a 92% sensitivity and negative predictive value [11]. For example, NICE type I lesions are hyperplastic, type II are adenomatous, and type III are concerning for containing deep submucosal cancer [11].

Work by Moss and colleagues has also found that polyps with Paris 0-II a-c morphology, non-granular surface and Kudo pit pattern V were at high risk for submucosal invasion [12]. Additionally, the NICE criteria have a 92% sensitivity and negative predictive value for prediction of submucosal carcinoma [11]. Type 3 lesions are associated with submucosal invasion.

The non-lifting sign is an indicator if the surrounding submucosal tissue lifts, but the lesion does not with injection. Lesions may not lift due to submucosal invasion or because of submucosal fibrosis from prior biopsy, cautery, or tattoo (Fig. 5.1). Studies have demonstrated that the presence of the non-lifting sign is associated with a positive predictive value for invasive cancer to be approximately 80% [13]. Additional signs of submucosal invasion include converging folds, chicken skin appearance, expansive appearance, and firm consistency [14].

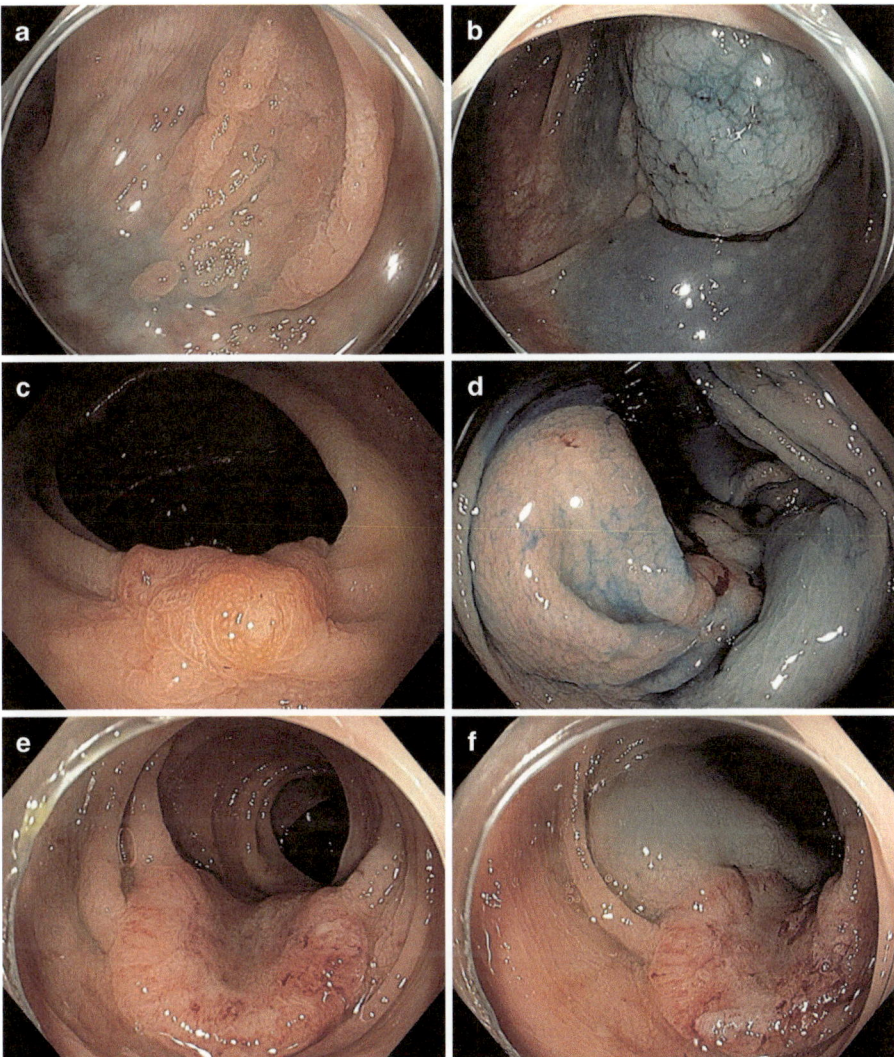

Fig. 5.1 The non-lifting sign

5.3   Resection Technique

Advanced endoscopic techniques include the standard inject-and-cut endoscopic mucosal resection (EMR) as well as endoscopic submucosal dissection (ESD). Adjunctive EMR techniques such as EMR with cap, underwater EMR, and EMR with cold snare have been more recently applied and studied. En bloc or R0 resection is ideal, though in lesions >20 mm this may not be feasible, and the goal should be to remove the lesion in as few pieces as safely possible.

5.3.1 Instruments and Equipment

Personnel should have familiarity with the range of equipment used and the technical aspects of the procedure. We recommend the use of a high-definition adult colonoscope with a water-jet channel and CO_2 insufflation in most cases. A therapeutic upper endoscope may be an alternative for left-colon lesions. Additionally, we prefer the use of conscious sedation over deep sedation with propofol [14].

5.4 EMR Techniques

5.4.1 Inject-and-Cut

The inject-and-cut EMR is a simple technique that is widely used for removal of large flat or sessile lesions. Submucosal injection is a key step of EMR. In this technique, saline is injected into the submucosal space of the colon wall. Injection in the submucosal layer is first confirmed using a small amount of solution, followed by rapid large-volume injection. We recommend the use of the dynamic injection technique to create a sufficient bleb under the lesion (Fig. 5.2). Unlike in static injection, the tip of the endoscope is slightly directed to the opposite wall coupled with a slight pull back of the needle catheter and simultaneous gentle suctioning [15]. Using this maneuver, the needle tip is maintained in the superficial submucosa, and a localized bleb can be easily created. This mound of fluid creates a cushion for resection as well as brings the lesion into the lumen toward the colonoscope.

Saline is the most commonly used solution though it may quickly dissipate. Viscous solutions such as hydroxyethyl starch, sodium hyaluronate solution, 50% dextrose, and succinylated gelatin are alternatives to improve maintenance of submucosal cushion. A 2016 systematic review compared normal saline to sodium hyaluronate, 50% dextrose,

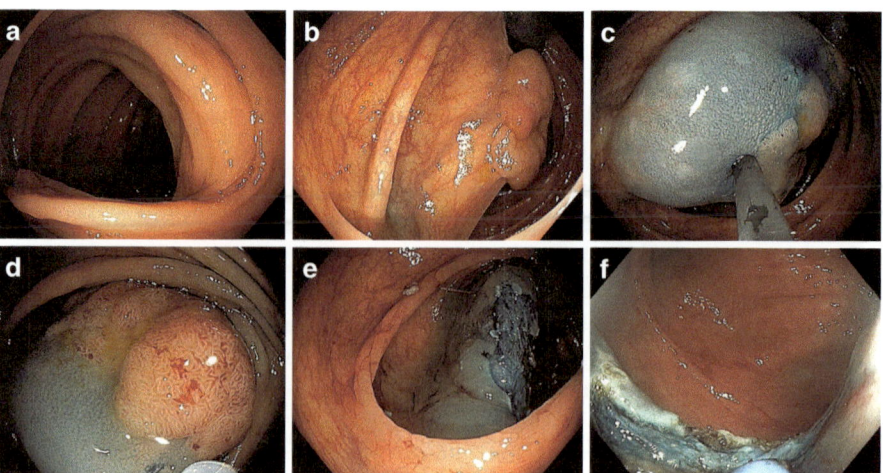

Fig. 5.2 Dynamic submucosal injection

hydroxyethyl starch, and fibrinogen and found no difference in complete resection (OR 1.09, CI 0.82–1.45) and only limited data on the efficacy of the other viscous solutions [16]. A 2017 systematic review pooled the results of viscous solution and found that viscous solution increased en bloc resection (OR 1.91, CI 1.11–3.29) and decreased risk of residual lesions (OR 0.54, CI 0.32–0.91) compared to normal saline [17]. Therefore, if available, the use of viscous solutions should be considered. Succinylated gelatin is not available in the USA. Sodium hyaluronate, the most studied solution in three randomized controlled trials, is relatively expensive.

A stiff snare can then be used to capture the lesion of interest to perform EMR. After snare capturing of the lesion, carbon dioxide insufflation will expand the wall, and slight loosening of the snare with up tip deflection will release any entrapped muscularis propria. The snare is then closed entirely almost to the hub, and the lesion is transected using electrosurgical current (ERBE, Endocut Q Effect 3, Duration 1, Interval 4) [14]). Microprocessor control units use alternate cycles of short-cutting bursts with interval periods of coagulation and limit peak voltage with impedance feedback (Figs. 5.3 and 5.4).

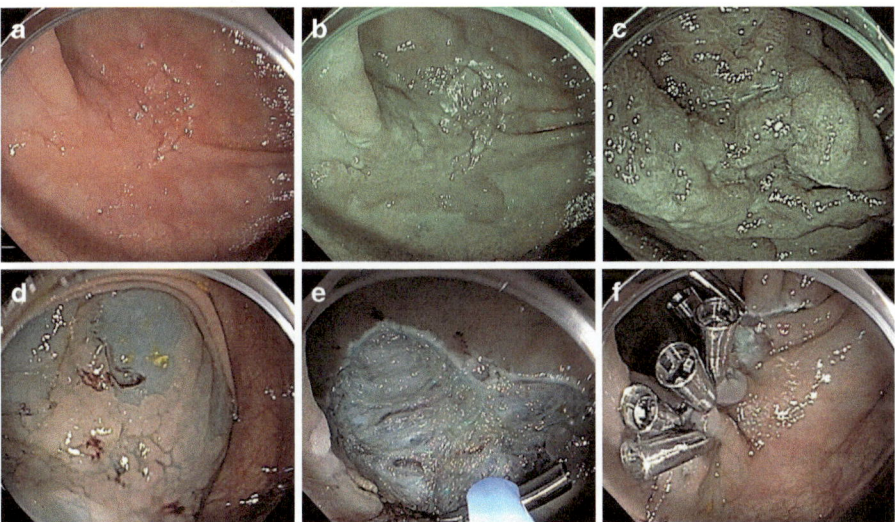

Fig. 5.3 Inject and cut endoscopic mucosal resection of nongranular lateral spreading lesion

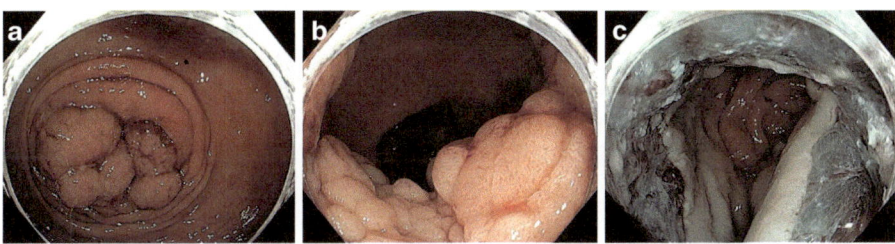

Fig. 5.4 Inject and cut endoscopic mucosal resection of granular lateral spreading lesion.

All visible neoplastic tissue should be resected in a single session. For lesions <20 mm, en bloc resection is recommended, particularly for LSL-NG lesions. Piecemeal EMR may be necessary for lesions larger than 20 mm. Due to the risk of submucosal invasion in the dominant nodule in an LSL-G, the dominant nodule should be resected and submitted to pathology separately. Ablative techniques, such as the use of snare tip soft coagulation and argon plasma coagulation (APC) on residual tissue, have been associated with an increased risk of local recurrence [18]. Once all neoplastic tissue has been removed, data suggests lower local recurrence rates when ablative therapies, such as APC or snare tip soft coagulation, are applied to the resection margin. A recent randomized controlled trial applying the snare tip in the soft coagulation mode to the defect periphery and bridges showed a significant reduction in recurrence rates. Recurrence outcomes using argon plasma coagulation versus snare tip soft coagulation have not been compared.

5.5 Alternative EMR Techniques

5.5.1 Cap-Assisted EMR

The use of a plastic cap during EMR can be useful to help deflect surrounding tissue during standard inject-and-cut EMR. Dedicated cap and snare devices can also be used for cap-assisted EMR in the rectum. Neoplastic tissue is suctioned into the cap, which can then be snared.

5.5.2 Underwater EMR

Underwater EMR was first described by Binmoeller et al. [19]. In underwater EMR, the water substitutes air insufflation. Injection is not necessary making this an alternative for fibrotic lesions. In his initial study of 60 patients, Binmoeller and colleagues demonstrated that the technique was safe with no perforation or post-polypectomy syndrome. Follow-up study by Curcio and colleagues in 2014 demonstrated complete resection at 3 months' follow-up in an additional 72 patients [20].

5.6 Cold Snare EMR

Cold snare EMR, whereby no electrosurgical cautery is applied, has been demonstrated to be feasible for lesions >1 cm. However, thus far evidence has been limited to single-center retrospective studies [21, 22].

5.7 ESD

Endoscopic submucosal dissection (ESD) is an alternative resection technique in the colon and particularly rectum. It is a technique mainly considered for complex lesions such as non-granular-type lateral spreading lesions with Vi pit pattern or those with concern for adenocarcinoma, with underlying fibrosis or with residual lesion after prior incomplete resection attempts (Table 5.1). Compared to EMR, ESD allows for en bloc resection of lesions (79% versus 34%); however, there is a higher risk of perforation (4.9% versus 0.9%) and need for surgery (7.8% versus 3.0%) [23] and significantly longer procedure time. Several studies have shown the safety and efficacy of EMR in the management of complex colorectal lesions, including those of large size, granular- and non-granular-type lateral spreading lesion morphology, and sessile serrated polyp histology [24].

5.7.1 Technique

ESD begins with marking the normal mucosa surrounding the lesion. Submucosal injection is then done to lift the lesion. The circumference of the lesion is then incised using a needle-type ESD knife, and the submucosal layer is then dissected. The resected en bloc can then be pinned and submitted to pathology. Attempts to simplify ESD technique have been described such as "precutting EMR," whereby the circumference of the lesion alone is incised by using a knife for ESD, and then the lesion is snared without submucosal dissection. Likewise, hybrid ESD is a technique in which an ESD knife dissects some of the submucosal layer, and then the lesion is snared (Fig. 5.5).

Table 5.1 Indications for ESD for colorectal tumors[a]

Lesions for which endoscopic en bloc resection is required
1. Lesions for which en bloc resection with snare EMR is difficult to apply
    • LST-NG, particularly LST-NG (PD)
    • Lesions showing a VI-type pit pattern
    • Carcinoma with shallow T1 (SM) invasion
    • Large depressed-type tumors
    • Large protruded-type lesions suspected to be carcinoma[b]
2. Mucosal tumors with submucosal fibrosis
3. Sporadic localized tumors in conditions of chronic inflammation such as ulcerative colitis
4. Local residual or recurrent early carcinomas after endoscopic resection

EMR endoscopic mucosal resection, *ESD* endoscopic submucosal dissection, *LST-G* laterally spreading tumor granular type, *LST-NG* laterally spreading tumor non-granular type, *PD* pseudo-depressed, *SM* submucosal
Tanaka S, Kashida H, Saito Y et al. JGES guidelines for colorectal endoscopic submucosal dissection/endoscopic mucosal resection Digestive Endoscopy 2015
[a]Partially modified from the draft proposed by the Colorectal ESD. Standardization implementation working group
[b]Including LST-G, nodular mixed type

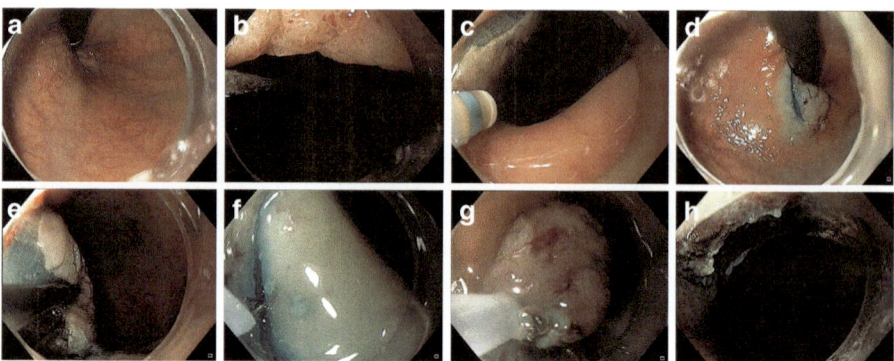

Fig. 5.5 Hybrid ESD of rectal lesion

5.8 Special Considerations

5.8.1 Scar

Previous treatment, such as biopsy, snaring, EMR, or tattoo, can cause submucosal scarring. Submucosal injection may be ineffective in formation of a submucosal bleb. The lesion may be difficult to snare, and inadvertent slippage of the snare can lead to perforation. Furthermore, pathology of the scarred tissue may be difficult to interpret. Avulsion of scarred or residual neoplastic tissue with biopsy forceps and high-frequency cutting current is a recently promising method for non-lifting tissue that is difficult to capture and resect using a snare [25]. A single-center retrospective study showed significantly lower recurrence rate in such non-lifting areas using hot avulsion compared to APC (OR 0.079, $p < 0.001$) [26].

5.8.2 Pedunculated Polyps

Pedunculated polyps are supplied by multiple blood vessels, and resection should take into account reducing the risk of bleeding. Options include the use of a detachable snare (Endoloop), clipping, or epinephrine injection to ligate the vasculature in the stalk of the pedunculated polyp. A randomized control trial in 2004 compared epinephrine injection versus detachable snare and found that both significantly decreased the risk of bleeding from 15.1% to 2.7% and 2.9%, respectively, but that there was no significant difference between epinephrine injection and detachable snare [27]. Whereas studies have shown a 5.4% risk of bleeding with hemoclip use [28].

Regardless of technique, the patient should be positioned, so the polyp attaches at the 12 o'clock position, and the colonoscope is rotated, so the stalk is at the 6 o'clock position. The endoloop or clips should be placed at the stalk so that the lesion turns dark red indicating that the polyp has been appropriately strangulated. Snare resection can then take place. Epinephrine has been described for polyp size reduction. It is to be injected into the head of the polyp to reduce polyp volume and allow for snaring. This may take up to 8 mL of 1:10,000 epinephrine [14].

5.9   Complications

The most common complications after endoscopic resection include bleeding and perforation.

The risk of perforation after EMR is 1–2% and 5–10% after ESD. Delayed perforation is thought to result from mural injury at the time of resection and recognition at the time of resection can decrease the risk of mortality and need for surgery. The target sign, the appearance of a white central circular disk representing the muscularis propria, surrounded by stained submucosa and a white cauterized, is an early indication of perforation [29]. More subtle signs of deep mucosal injury include focal loss of the submucosal plane raising concern MP injury. Prophylactic clipping is recommended to prevent clinically significant perforation [30].

Bleeding after endoscopic resection can occur immediately or be delayed. There is a 7–9% risk of bleeding after endoscopic resection [3]. Various methods such as soft-tip snare coagulation, coagulation forceps, or clip can be used to treat immediate bleeding at the time of resection. A 2014 study found that clinically significant post-endoscopic bleeding as defined by emergency department visit, hospitalization, or need for intervention occurs after 6.3% of EMRs for lesions >20 mm and is associated with proximal colon location, the use of electrosurgical cautery without a microprocessor unit but not lesion size, or comorbidities [31]. Fifty-five percent of these bleeds resolved spontaneously, and only 33% required endoscopic therapy [32].

5.10   Recurrence and Surveillance

Risk of recurrence in EMR is higher than ESD and is estimated to be 16% at the initial colonoscopy and 4% late colonoscopy. Due to the risk of recurrence, careful surveillance is recommended. The initial follow-up endoscopic exam is recommended at 6 months. Risk factors for recurrence include LSL $\geq$ 40 mm, bleeding during procedure, and high-grade dysplasia. Tate and colleagues proposed the Sydney EMR recurrence tool (SERT) scoring system based on these risk factors and suggest that those with a SERT score of 1 or more should have surveillance at 6 and 18 months, whereas those with a SERT score of 0 could safely undergo first surveillance at 18 months [33].

We recommend standard performance of surveillance colonoscopy at 6 months with a high-definition colonoscope. Careful inspection of the scar should be performed with white light and NBI to assess for evidence of macroscopic recurrence.

A prospective single-center study found that white light with NBI has a 94% (CI 89.6–99.6%) accuracy compared to 91.3% (86.3–94.6%) with white light alone [34]. Biopsies should be taken of the scar site even if no macroscopic recurrence is detected. We recommend repeat EMR or ESD for recurrence and continued surveillance at 6 month until clear and then 1 year and then 3 years.

Conclusion
Endoscopic resection should be the treatment of choice for complex colon polyps. Advanced resection techniques should be used to safely accomplish resection of such lesions. Complications of perforation and bleeding should be recognized and can be managed endoscopically. Continued surveillance with colonoscopy at 6 months after index procedure is important to detect and treat recurrences.

References

1. Raju GS, Lum PJ, Ross WA, et al. Outcome of EMR as an alternative to surgery in patients with complex colon polyps. Gastrointest Endosc. 2016;84:315–25.
2. Law R, Das A, Gregory D, et al. Endoscopic resection is cost-effective compared with laparoscopic resection in the management of complex colon polyps: an economic analysis. Gastrointest Endosc. 2016;83:1248–57.
3. Hassan C, Repici A, Sharma P, et al. Efficacy and safety of endoscopic resection of large colorectal polyps: a systematic review and meta-analysis. Gut. 2016;65:806–20.
4. The Paris endoscopic classification of superficial neoplastic lesions: esophagus, stomach, and colon: November 30 to December 1, 2002. Gastrointest Endosc. 2003;58:S3–43.
5. Endoscopic Classification Review Group. Update on the paris classification of superficial neoplastic lesions in the digestive tract. Endoscopy. 2005;37:570–8.
6. Kudo S, Lambert R, Allen JI, et al. Nonpolypoid neoplastic lesions of the colorectal mucosa. Gastrointest Endosc. 2008;68:S3–47.
7. Soetikno RM, Kaltenbach T, Rouse RV, et al. Prevalence of nonpolypoid (flat and depressed) colorectal neoplasms in asymptomatic and symptomatic adults. JAMA. 2008;299:1027–35.
8. Kudo SE, Kashida H. Flat and depressed lesions of the colorectum. Clin Gastroenterol Hepatol. 2005;3:S33–6.
9. McGill SK, Evangelou E, Ioannidis JP, et al. Narrow band imaging to differentiate neoplastic and non-neoplastic colorectal polyps in real time: a meta-analysis of diagnostic operating characteristics. Gut. 2013;62:1704–13.
10. Kudo S, Tamura S, Nakajima T, et al. Diagnosis of colorectal tumorous lesions by magnifying endoscopy. Gastrointest Endosc. 1996;44:8–14.
11. Hayashi N, Tanaka S, Hewett DG, et al. Endoscopic prediction of deep submucosal invasive carcinoma: validation of the narrow-band imaging international colorectal endoscopic (NICE) classification. Gastrointest Endosc. 2013;78:625–32.
12. Moss A, Bourke MJ, Williams SJ, et al. Endoscopic mucosal resection outcomes and prediction of submucosal cancer from advanced colonic mucosal neoplasia. Gastroenterology. 2011;140:1909–18.
13. Kobayashi N, Saito Y, Sano Y, et al. Determining the treatment strategy for colorectal neoplastic lesions: endoscopic assessment or the non-lifting sign for diagnosing invasion depth? Endoscopy. 2007;39:701–5.
14. Sanchez-Yague A, Kaltenbach T, Raju G, et al. Advanced endoscopic resection of colorectal lesions. Gastroenterol Clin N Am. 2013;42:459–77.

15. Soetikno R, Kaltenbach T. Dynamic submucosal injection technique. Gastrointest Endosc Clin N Am. 2010;20:497–502.
16. Ferreira AO, Moleiro J, Torres J, et al. Solutions for submucosal injection in endoscopic resection: a systematic review and meta-analysis. Endosc Int Open. 2016;4:E1–E16.
17. Yandrapu H, Desai M, Siddique S, et al. Normal saline solution versus other viscous solutions for submucosal injection during endoscopic mucosal resection: a systematic review and meta-analysis. Gastrointest Endosc. 2017;85:693–9.
18. Moss A, Williams SJ, Hourigan LF, et al. Long-term adenoma recurrence following wide-field endoscopic mucosal resection (WF-EMR) for advanced colonic mucosal neoplasia is infrequent: results and risk factors in 1000 cases from the Australian colonic EMR (ACE) study. Gut. 2015;64:57–65.
19. Binmoeller KF, Weilert F, Shah J, et al. "Underwater" EMR without submucosal injection for large sessile colorectal polyps (with video). Gastrointest Endosc. 2012;75:1086–91.
20. Curcio G, Granata A, Ligresti D, et al. Underwater colorectal EMR: remodeling endoscopic mucosal resection. Gastrointest Endosc. 2015;81:1238–42.
21. Piraka C, Saeed A, Waljee AK, et al. Cold snare polypectomy for non-pedunculated colon polyps greater than 1 cm. Endosc Int Open. 2017;5:E184–9.
22. Choksi N, Elmunzer BJ, Stidham RW, et al. Cold snare piecemeal resection of colonic and duodenal polyps >/=1 cm. Endosc Int Open. 2015;3:E508–13.
23. Arezzo A, Passera R, Marchese N, et al. Systematic review and meta-analysis of endoscopic submucosal dissection vs endoscopic mucosal resection for colorectal lesions. United European Gastroenterol J. 2016;4:18–29.
24. Rao AK, Soetikno R, Raju GS, et al. Large sessile serrated polyps can be safely and effectively removed by endoscopic mucosal resection. Clin Gastroenterol Hepatol. 2016;14:568–74.
25. Veerappan SG, Ormonde D, Yusoff IF, et al. Hot avulsion: a modification of an existing technique for management of nonlifting areas of a polyp (with video). Gastrointest Endosc. 2014;80:884–8.
26. Holmes I, Kim HG, Yang DH, et al. Avulsion is superior to argon plasma coagulation for treatment of visible residual neoplasia during EMR of colorectal polyps (with videos). Gastrointest Endosc. 2016;84:822–9.
27. Di Giorgio P, De Luca L, Calcagno G, et al. Detachable snare versus epinephrine injection in the prevention of postpolypectomy bleeding: a randomized and controlled study. Endoscopy. 2004;36:860–3.
28. Boo SJ, Byeon JS, Park SY, et al. Clipping for the prevention of immediate bleeding after polypectomy of pedunculated polyps: a pilot study. Clin Endosc. 2012;45:84–8.
29. Swan MP, Bourke MJ, Moss A, et al. The target sign: an endoscopic marker for the resection of the muscularis propria and potential perforation during colonic endoscopic mucosal resection. Gastrointest Endosc. 2011;73:79–85.
30. Ma MX, Bourke MJ. Complications of endoscopic polypectomy, endoscopic mucosal resection and endoscopic submucosal dissection in the colon. Best Pract Res Clin Gastroenterol. 2016;30:749–67.
31. Burgess NG, Metz AJ, Williams SJ, et al. Risk factors for intraprocedural and clinically significant delayed bleeding after wide-field endoscopic mucosal resection of large colonic lesions. Clin Gastroenterol Hepatol. 2014;12:651–61. e1-3
32. Burgess NG, Williams SJ, Hourigan LF, et al. A management algorithm based on delayed bleeding after wide-field endoscopic mucosal resection of large colonic lesions. Clin Gastroenterol Hepatol. 2014;12:1525–33.
33. Tate DJ, Desomer L, Klein A, et al. Adenoma recurrence after piecemeal colonic EMR is predictable: the Sydney EMR recurrence tool. Gastrointest Endosc. 2017;85:647–56. e6
34. Desomer L, Tutticci N, Tate DJ, et al. A standardized imaging protocol is accurate in detecting recurrence after EMR. Gastrointest Endosc. 2017;85:518–26.

Colorectal Endoscopic Submucosal Dissection

6

Federico Iacopini and Yutaka Saito

6.1 Introduction

Colorectal carcinoma is the most common gastrointestinal cancer and the third most frequently diagnosed malignancy in adults. Screening for colorectal cancer reduces the incidence [1] and mortality [2] through the detection and removal of adenomatous polyps and early stage cancers. The 5-year survival rate of colorectal carcinoma was reported to be 94% for stage 0 and 91% for stage I after surgery and 93% after endoscopic resection. Given that endotherapy is less morbid and less expensive than surgery [3], it should be considered as the first line of treatment of early colorectal carcinomas with little possibility of lymph node metastasis based on histologic features (microstaging): cancer differentiation well or moderate, submucosal (SM) invasion depth <1000 μm (T1a), lymphovascular invasion negative, and budding grade 1 [4, 5].

Various techniques in endoscopic resection can be selected and basically, en bloc resection would be the gold standard [6–10]. Endoscopic mucosal resection (EMR) is efficient, utilizes not expensive equipments, has a low perforation rate (<1%), and can be performed in an outpatient setting as a day stay case, enhancing convenience for patients and significantly reducing costs. However, neoplasms >20 mm are resected in multiple pieces (piecemeal EMR) with a high rate of incomplete resection and recurrence (up to 20% in recent studies), a difficult histologic microstaging and free resection margin determination. Accordingly, endoscopic submucosal dissection (ESD) was pioneered in Japan in the late 1990s as a better alternative for the removal of early gastric cancers. ESD has the ability to

F. Iacopini
Gastroenterology Endoscopy Unit, S. Giuseppe Hospital, Albano L., Rome, Italy

Y. Saito (✉)
Endoscopy Division, National Cancer Center Hospital,
5-1-1 Tsukiji, Chuo-ku, Tokyo 104-0045, Japan
e-mail: ytsaito@ncc.go.jp

© Springer International Publishing AG 2018
A. Facciorusso, N. Muscatiello (eds.), *Colon Polypectomy*,
https://doi.org/10.1007/978-3-319-59457-6_6

resect lesions en bloc regardless of their size and achieve accurate histological evaluation, decreasing recurrence and increasing cure rates. In a meta-analysis including 14 studies, Puli et al. [11] concluded that ESD is the best endoscopic technique and an alternative to surgery. Nowadays, ESD has become the therapeutic modality of choice for superficial cancers both in the upper and lower gastrointestinal tract in Japan and East Asia bringing a renaissance of therapeutic endoscopy and offering an organ-sparing cure [12]. However, ESD is performed by only in a handful of Western endoscopists and EMR remains the standard [5]. In the West, the adoption of ESD for all superficial colorectal neoplasms >20 mm is considered premature since the majority of lesions are benign adenoma and colorectal ESD is complex and requires long operating time and increased resource utilization, and there is not an adequate reimbursement. Finally, the main obstacle for ESD adoption in the West is the very flat learning curve and the lack of a training protocol [13].

6.2   Indications

An accurate diagnosis directed both to assess the risk of malignancy of the lesion and identify its carcinomatous areas is essential to select the endoscopic approach [14, 15]. Neoplasm characterization and ESD adoption would probably change the yield of the local excision in the natural history of superficial neoplasms. The indications for the en bloc resection have been identified by the colorectal ESD standardization implementation working group (Table 6.1) [4]. Neoplasms candidate to ESD can be differentiated in two classes: (1) those suspected of being slightly invasive into the SM and (2) those with SM fibrosis.

Criteria of the first class are based on recent strong evidences. The risk and the depth of SM invasion can be accurately predicted according to neoplasm morphology and superficial patterns (endoscopic characterization). Neoplasms with slight SM invasion not precluding a curative endoscopic resection should be removed en bloc to accurately evaluate all histologic features prognostic of LN metastasis.

Table 6.1 Indications by colorectal ESD standardization implementation working group

Neoplasms suspected of slightly SM invasion	Large-sized (>20 mm) lesions in which en bloc resection by EMR is difficult
	LST-NG, particularly those of the pseudo-depressed type
	Lesions showing V_I-type pit pattern
	Carcinoma with SM infiltration
	Large depressed-type lesion
	Large elevated lesion suspected to be carcinoma (LST-G nodular mixed type and sessile polyps)
Neoplasms with SM fibrosis	Mucosal lesions with fibrosis caused by prolapse due to biopsy or peristalsis of the lesions
	Sporadic localized tumors in chronic inflammation (such as ulcerative colitis)
	Local residual early carcinoma after endoscopic resection

The first step of characterization is the evaluation of the neoplasm morphology. A recent study from the National Cancer Center Hospital (NCCH) in Tokyo was based on the histologic analysis of the largest series of colorectal neoplasms removed en bloc by endoscopy or surgery. This study confirms their previous data [16] and provides new insights. Laterally spreading tumors with a granular surface (LST-G) showed an SM invasion in 19% (80/414) of cases, which was localized under a nodule >10 mm in 56% (n.45), a depressed area in 28% (n.22), or was multifocal in 16% (n.13). A deep SM invasion accounted for 79% (63/80) of invasive LST-Gs and was predicted by an invasive pit pattern in only 41% (n.33), with a sensibility of 80% in depressed areas, 43% under the nodule, and 17% in multifocal cases. Thus, it is clinically important to identify depressed areas and large nodules before endoscopic resection since the estimation of the SM invasion depth can be inaccurate: overall sensitivity of V_I (invasive)/V_N pit pattern being low (52%, 33/63) (Figs. 6.1, 6.2, and 6.3).

The same study showed that laterally spreading tumor with a nongranular surface (LST-NG) has a 39% prevalence of SM invasion (159/408), which is almost double than that of LST-G. This finding agrees with previous data [17, 18] and confirms that en bloc resection is mandatory for LST-NG. SM invasion was

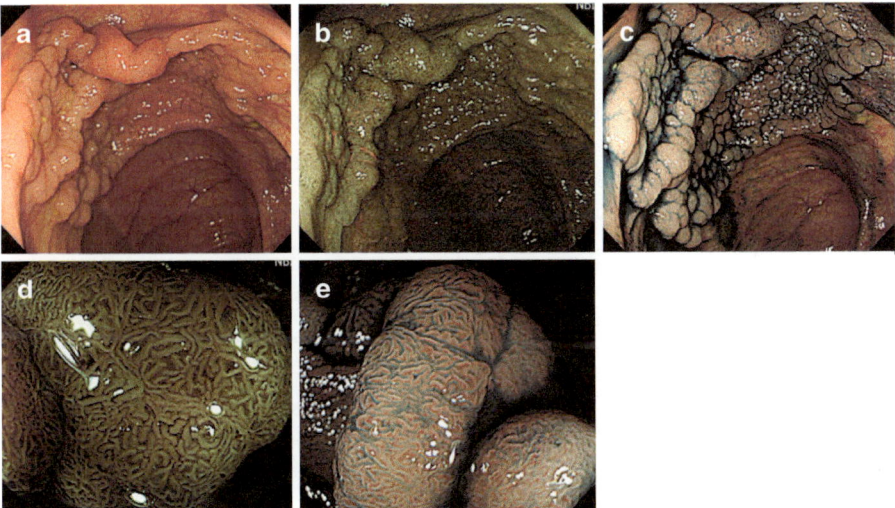

Fig. 6.1 (**a**) *White light* image revealed a large laterally spreading tumor granular type (LST-G) located in the cecum. (**b**) *Narrow band* imaging (NBI) image revealed a tumor boundary clearly, which was even more clear after indigo carmine spraying (**c**). (**d**) NBI with magnification revealed a regular vessel pattern and regular surface pattern suggesting Japan NBI Expert Team (JNET) type 2A. JNET type 2A corresponds to low-grade dysplasia in the West and adenoma or low-grade intramucosal cancer in Japan. (**e**) Indigo carmine dye spray with magnification revealed type IV and IIIL pit pattern corresponding to JNET type 2A. Final diagnosis of this tumor was LST-G nodular mixed type, 5 cm in diameter; the estimated histology was tubular adenoma or intramucosal cancer corresponding to low-grade intramucosal neoplasia in the West. Probably, piecemeal EMR (p-EMR) would be planned for this tumor in the West; however, an en bloc resection by ESD was performed at the NCCH, Tokyo, Japan

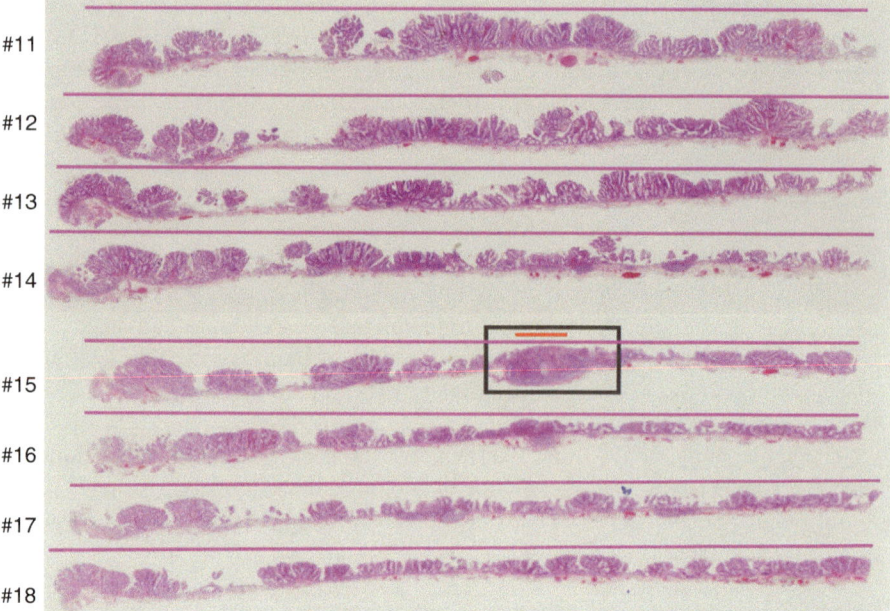

Fig. 6.2 Histology of the LST-G in Fig. 6.1: intramucosal cancer in most section. However, submucosal (SM) deep invasion was observed in one section of #15

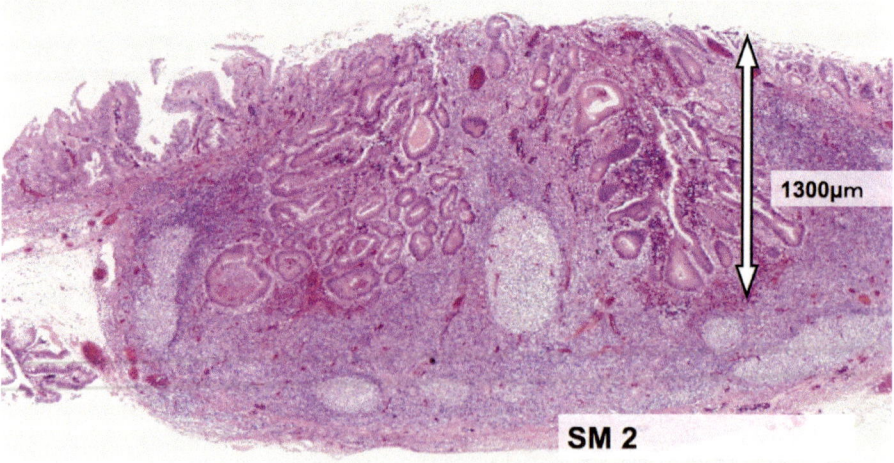

Fig. 6.3 High-power view of the section #15 (Fig. 6.2) revealed SM deep invasion. The muscularis mucosa was destroyed around this area; therefore, the invasion depth was measured from the tumor surface, and 1300 μm invasion was diagnosed. The cancer invasion deeper than 1000 μm was one of the risk factors for lymph node metastasis (LNM); consequently, an ileocecal resection with LN dissection was conducted

localized under a depressed area in 45% (n.71) and a SM mass in 10% (n.16), but was multifocal in 45% (n.72) cases. The SM invasion was deep in 54% of invasive LST-NG (86/151) and predicted by an invasive pattern in 71%: 83% under the SM mass, 68% in depressed areas, and 73% when multifocal. Pit pattern diagnosis was useful in estimating the SM depth of invasion in LST-NG.

The need of an en bloc resection for other colorectal neoplasm morphologies is more defined. Kudo et al. [19, 20] reported that the SM invasion of depressed lesions was 44% for lesions 6–10 mm and 89% (31/35) for lesions >15 mm. Sessile polyps showed a risk of SM invasion in 30% of lesions >20 mm [21].

The second step of characterization is based on the analysis of superficial pit and microvascular patterns to predict SM invasion depth and the risk of lymph node metastasis. Pit patterns are categorized according to the Kudo classification [22], whereas microvascular patterns should be defined according to the new classification proposed by the Japanese NBI Expert Team (JNET), which has with important clinical implications [23]. A detailed determination of the type V (irregular) pit pattern by magnifying chromoendoscopy, its differentiation in type V_I and V_N, and the further stratification of type V_I in slightly and highly irregular is important to predict the rate of deep SM invasion: 6–11% in slightly irregular V_I, 49–56% in highly irregular V_I, and 96% in V_N [24, 25].

The second class of neoplasms for which ESD is indicated comprises lesions whose main feature is SM fibrosis and poor lifting either related to luminal prolapse/peristalsis, scars of previous attempts of resection (or biopsies and tattoos), or chronic inflammatory conditions (i.e., inflammatory bowel diseases, IBD). These lesions are the most challenging showing a high failure and incomplete EMR even using stiff snares. Although experience is a major determinant for the success [26], alternative techniques have been proposed for a complete resection: hot avulsion for small remnants (mean size 4.4 mm [27], ablation by argon plasma coagulation for larger remnants with the disadvantage of the lack of histology [28]. A hybrid EMR/ESD approach based on a partial SM dissection and the use of the snare was found to achieve a 38% en bloc resection rate, a 35% complete resection in more than one session, and a 16% recurrence rate [29]. In this context, ESD shows better outcomes even when the lesion is >20 mm: en bloc resection ranged from 56 to 93%; recurrence rate was 0% [30–32]. However, ESD has been evaluated in small case series and the procedure is significantly more difficult than in naïve lesions with a high risk of perforation (15% vs. 4%) [32]. These data indicate that experts should attempt ESD of residual/scarring neoplasms.

Peculiar neoplasms for which en bloc resection by ESD has been proposed are large non-polypoid lesions in IBD. Prophylactic proctocolectomy traditionally advocated to treat these neoplasms has been substituted by endoscopic resection if a curative (en bloc) excision can be achieved and adjacent mucosa is normal [33]. EMR is inadequate in this setting due to inadequate lesion lifting secondary to the chronic long-standing mucosa/submucosal inflammation [34]. Efficacy of ESD for IBD non-polypoid neoplasms was evaluated in one cooperative Italian and Japanese study on a small number of cases [35]. This study demonstrated that ESD might expand the curative purposes of endoscopy in long-standing ulcerative colitis avoiding unnecessary surgery. Despite a very high (90%) prevalence of SM fibrosis, the en bloc and R0 resection rate was 80%, and the perforation rate was 0%.

6.2.1 Colorectal ESD vs. Piecemeal EMR

Piecemeal EMR has proven to be an excellent treatment in expert hands and represents the standard for most of the lesions in the West [18, 26]. Curative resections of large adenomas and carcinoma in situ can be achieved by EMR if the number of resected pieces is minimized and the region suspected to contain a carcinoma is not sectioned [14, 16, 36]. Conversely, piecemeal EMR is today almost never intentionally performed in Japan and East Asia. Japan is the ESD cradle: the procedure was introduced to treat early gastric cancer, progressively applied in all GI segments, and indications have been proposed and standardized [4].

ESD and EMR have been compared in many nonrandomized studies and meta-analyses. One of the most recent meta-analysis by Puli et al. [11] showed that the outcomes (pooled odds ratios, OR, [95% confidence interval]) of ESD were superior to those of EMR for en bloc resection (6.84 [3.30–14.18]), curative resection (4.26 [3.77–6.57]), and recurrence (0.08 [0.04–0.17]), even if neoplasms were significantly larger (7.38 [6.42–8.34]). Conversely, ESD required significantly longer operating time (58.07 [36.27–79.88]) and was associated with a higher risk of perforation (4.96 [2.79–8.85]). The significantly higher rate of additional surgery in the ESD group (2.16 [1.16–4.03]) was mainly related to a higher rate of invasive neoplasms rather to perforation. The higher efficacy of ESD than EMR for lesions >20 mm has been also confirmed in prospective multicenter studies from expert Western and Japanese centers (Table 6.2).

Table 6.2 Outcomes of EMR and ESD for superficial colorectal neoplasms >20 mm from prospective studies conducted by two expert centers from Japan and Western countries

	Moss [18]	Nakajima [37] Oka [38]*	
Study design	Multicenter (n.7) prospective	Multicenter (n.18) prospective	
Technique	EMR	EMR	ESD
n. procedures	514	1029	816
Neoplasm size, mm (median [range])	36 (20–100)	26 (20–120)	39 (20–174)
En bloc (%)	n.a. (4 pieces/lesion)	55	95
Procedure time (min) (mean [SD])	25 (22)	18 (23)	96 (69)
Perforation (%)	1.3	0.8	2
Recurrence (%)	27	6.8*	1.4*

*Data from Oka [38]

6.3 Training

A standardized training protocol has been identified in Japan and makes ESD widely available in the national health system. This is not true in the West due to the low gastric cancer incidence and working environment. Trainees embarking on ESD in the West differ significantly from their Eastern counterparts: a GI fellow in Japan and a mature otherwise experienced therapeutic endoscopist in the West. However, the ESD training should be based on the sequential achievement of different skills differentiated in three phases.

6.3.1 Propaedeutic Skills

ESD trainees should be experts in colonoscopy, neoplasia characterization, and therapeutic interventions. Colonoscopy should be performed with high cecal intubation rates and no loops so to reach the neoplasm with a straight scope and finely control the tip movements. Characterization of the risk and depth of SM invasion is mandatory to choose the appropriate resection approach. Endoscopists should be familiar with EMR and should know how to conduct and control the depth of cut, a resection above semilunar folds, and recognize the muscle layer and its injuries. Intraoperative bleeding is common during ESD but should not be considered as an adverse event. However, it needs to be promptly and systematically controlled and prevented since it significantly increases the procedure difficulty. A competence in hemostasis and clip placement prior to starting performing ESD is required [39, 40]. The relevance of other therapeutic skills remains uncertain. Finally, the ESD trainee should also have some aptitudes: perseverance, competence in dealing with stressful situations, and awareness of own limitations.

6.3.2 Theoretic Phase

A solid cognitive preparation is the basis for training. The trainee should be aware of the ESD technique, specific approaches for each GI segment, mechanical properties and maneuverability of endoscopes, working plan of each dissecting knife, management of minor and major adverse events, specimen fixation and pathological assessment, and postoperative surveillance.

Japanese and Western training protocols begin to differ in this phase. Japanese trainees learn ESD in high-volume expert centers while observing and serving as assistants. Westerns have to rely on workshops, lives demonstrations, and online materials. However, expert observation is irreplaceable, and a visit to expert centers represents a great advantage. Although being not allowed to be involved in interventions, doctors visiting high-volume expert centers observe a huge number of procedures performed both by experts and trainees covering the whole spectrum of situations. Moreover, they may practice in animal models with the unique opportunity of supervision [41].

6.3.3 Hands-On Phase

Differences between Japan and the West increase widely in this phase. Japanese trainees generally follow a stepwise approach based on an increase of ESD difficulty moving from the distal gastric antrum, to the gastric body and cardia, up to the esophagus and colon. These steps are made under the supervision of experts or senior endoscopists who offers advices and complete the procedure if necessary.

Gastric ESD (g-ESD) represents the first step. The large lumen facilitates the approach, and the thick wall decreases the risk of perforation [42, 43]. A median of 30 g-ESDs is required for the self-competition of the procedure in the antrum [44, 45], but 40 and 80 procedures would be the minimum for a proficiency in the middle and upper thirds of the stomach [46] and an expertise level, respectively [40, 47]. Colorectal ESD (cr-ESD) is allowed after the achievement of g-ESD competence. The colon has a narrow windy lumen, folds, and a thinner wall. Thus, the procedure is significantly more difficult and the risk of perforation and peritonitis is higher. The learning curve for cr-ESD has been analyzed in several Japanese studies starting from the g-ESD experience (Table 6.3). Sakamoto et al. [48] at the NCCH reported that a basic competence is reached after 30 cr-ESDs. Other Japanese authors reported that the threshold for competency may range from 10 to 40 procedures, and 80 cr-ESDs could be required to achieve an expertise level [49].

The need of a propaedeutic competence in the stomach and expert supervision limits the adoption of this protocol in the West. The low incidence of gastric cancer and the low proportion of early lesions diagnosed during upper endoscopy [53] reduce the opportunity to start in easier locations, whereas a

Table 6.3 Learning curves in colorectal ESD based on a previous experience typical of the Japanese setting

	Operator		CR-ESD competence	
	n., supervision	Previous experience	Threshold (proc. n.)	Measures
Hotta [49]	1, yes	g-ESD (n. 20)	40	Op. speed: signif. increase Perforation: 12% to 5%
Sakamoto [48]	2, yes	g-ESD (n. >20) cr-ESD assistance	30	Self-completion: 45% to 92% Perforation: 5% (no change)
Probst [50]	2, no	g-ESD (n.150) e-ESD (n.40)	25	En bloc: 60% to 88%
Niimi [51]	1, yes	g-ESD (n. >30) cr-ESD assistance animal models	n.a.	En bloc: 91% Perforation: 4%
Shiga [52]	4, yes	g-ESD (n.5) cr-ESD assistance animal models	10	R0: 64% to 90% Perforation: 15% to 0%

g-ESD gastric ESD, *e-ESD* esophageal ESD, *cr-ESD* colorectal ESD

Table 6.4 Learning curves in colorectal ESD based on training protocols reproducible in the Western setting

| | Operator | | cr-ESD competence | |
	n., supervision	Previous experience	Threshold (proc. n.)	Measures
Iacopini [55]	1, no	Exp. observation Animal model (n.6)	r-ESD: n.20 c-ESD: n.20	En bloc: 60% to 80% En bloc: 20% to 80%
Yang [56]	1, on demand	Exp. observation CI-EMR	50	En bloc: 72% to 80% Perforation: 14% to 6% after 100

r-ESD rectal ESD, *c-ESD* colonic ESD, *CI-EMR* circumferential incision EMR

handful of highly qualified experts makes supervision impractical [54]. The Western unfavorable setting and the lack of a standard training protocol are probably the main reason to still considering EMR the best approach. However, alternative steps have been indicated in a recent European position statement based on Japanese expert recommendations: hands-on skills should be sought on animal models and then on antral and rectal lesions in humans [5, 13]. Compared to the colon, the rectum has a straight and larger lumen, fewer folds, and is wrapped by the mesorectal tissue that reduces the clinical relevance of a perforation reducing the risk of peritonitis. A small neoplasm in the lower rectum may be treatable as similar to that in the gastric antrum, whereas a lesion involving anal canal seems to be similar to one at the cardia. A stepwise training protocol based on the ESD competence in the rectum as propaedeutic to that in the colon has been investigated in one study conducted in Italy (Table 6.4) [55]. The single operator was expert in therapeutic endoscopy, had a limited ESD experience on ex vivo animal models, and visited the NCCH in Tokyo for a short period before practicing on humans. Competence in rectal and colonic ESD (defined as 80% en bloc rate plus significant reduction of operating speed) was safely achieved after 20 procedures in both locations. Another recent study from South Korea showed that a learning curve in cr-ESD can be started after an experience in hybrid ESD. The ESD en bloc resection rate increased to 80% after 50 procedures, and perforation rate decreased from 14% to 6% after 100 procedures (Table 6.4) [56].

6.3.4   Animal Models

Training on animal models is a feasible option for endoscopists in the West wishing to acquire ESD competency. A recent prospective Japanese study by Ohata et al. [57] demonstrated that the ex vivo porcine model provides sufficient experience to safely perform cr-ESD in humans. Six ESDs in an isolated colon significantly decreased the operating speed, and 12 procedures were sufficient to start cr-ESD with a 100% en bloc resection and 0–10% perforation. A positive impact of animal models on ESD training has been reported by other authors (Table 6.5).

Table 6.5 Learning curves in ESD on animal ex vivo models

	Previous experience	Animal model	ESD competence Threshold (proc. n.)	Measures
Hon [58]	None	Ex vivo porcine colon	n.a.	Op. time
Yoshida [59]	cr-ESD <10	Fresh ex vivo bovine & porcine colon	n.a.	Op. time
Kato [60]	None	Ex vivo porcine stomach	30	En bloc and perforation
Pioche [61]	Animal model: 6	Ex vivo bovine colon	16	Op. speed
Ohata [57]	None	Ex vivo porcine colon	6	Op. speed

Although these results may not be fully reproducible in the West since conducted under expert supervision, training on animal models seems to facilitate familiarity both with ESD tools and techniques and differences depending on neoplasm size and location. A basic experience on animal models should be recommended before starting in humans [39] to manage a risk of perforation that can rise up to 35% during the first cases [62].

6.4   Alternative Approaches

Hybridization of EMR and ESD may deliver substantial gains: increase in en bloc resection efficacy (decreased recurrence rate; more accurate histologic microstaging), improved feasibility with EMR competence, and utilization as intermediate steps in the hands-on ESD training phase. Hybrid resections differ according to the grade of hybridization of the two techniques and are defined as: CI-EMR when the circumferential incision of the mucosa is followed by snare resection; hybrid ESD when SM dissection is conducted up to a feasible en bloc snare resection.

Indications for CI-EMR and hybrid ESD rely on lesion size and probably lesion morphology. A prospective study on animal models from expert Australian authors suggested that CI-EMR could replace piecemeal EMR as the technique of choice for LST <40 mm with a 70% en bloc resection rate [63]. Results from a prospective study on humans conducted by Japanese experts were different: the en bloc resection by CI-EMR was suitable in almost all 20–30 mm lesions (94%) but in just few of those measuring 30–40 mm (6%) [64]. However, this study showed that CI-EMR achieved a complete resection in one or two pieces in 84% of cases, and the recurrence rate was 0%, much lower than the 10–26% reported when the specimen number ranges from 3 to 4 [38, 65, 66]. Similarly, two retrospective comparative studies from Japan and South Korea showed a progressive increase in the en bloc resection efficacy with an increasing grade of hybridization toward ESD: 62% by CI-EMR, 65–91% by hybrid ESD, and 97–99% by ESD [67, 68].

6.5   Technical Developments

ESD is traditionally based on the repetition of SM injection and dissection to guarantee a safe dissection of the lesion from the muscularis propria. This goal may be simplified by either using long-lasting solutions or adopting new devices or dissection strategies.

Japanese experts generally use glycerol (10% glycerol and 5% fructose in normal saline solution) and sodium hyaluronate acid (the most long-acting agent) [69]. The use of these agents has resulted in safer, easier, and more effective ESDs than using just normal saline. With the same purpose, various knives with a water jet function that permits both to inject and cut without tool exchanges have been introduced: Flush knife BT (Fujifilm, Tokyo, Japan); Jet B-knife (Zeon Medical, Tokyo, Japan); Splash needle (Pentax Medical, Tokyo, Japan); Hybrid knife (ERBE Elektromedizin, Tubingen, Germany); and Dual-jet (Olympus, Tokyo, Japan). These knives seem to decrease both procedure time and increase safety [70–73].

The pocket-creation method is a new strategy to overcome some of the ESD difficulties. The mucosal incision is not circumferential until the SM dissection is finished in a tunneling fashion and the creation of a "pocket." This strategy prolongs the duration of SM injection, stabilizes the endoscope position, and facilitates tissue traction. The pocket-creation method seems to make cr-ESD easier (faster) and more effective (higher en bloc resection rate) [74].

Another strategy for easier ESD is the traction method using clip-nylon in distal colorectum and S-O clip traction in any location. Methods to improve countertraction make colorectal ESD easier and faster [75, 76].

6.6   Colorectal ESD Prognostics of Difficulty

The recognition of prognostics of cr-ESD difficulty would improve both its feasibility and safety. This effort has been exclusively evaluated by Japanese authors with some discordance mainly due to different study designs, definitions of difficulty, and neoplasm features [52, 77–83]. The largest multicenter study conducted in Japan by Takeuchi et al. [82] showed that preoperative prognostics of difficulty were size >40 mm (OR 5), a poor scope operability (OR 2.8), and poor lesion lifting (OR 10.7). However, there were also intraoperative prognostics that contribute to the gradient of difficulty: scope operability, SM fibrosis, gravity, and countertraction efficacy [78, 81–83].

The definitive identification of prognostics of difficulty and/or severe adverse events and predicted gradients of difficulty would be the most effective intervention to boost a widespread cr-ESD adoption. Outcomes are susceptible to many different difficulties that cannot be fully addressed with the basic level of competency. A steady 85% en bloc resection rate and low perforation rate (<5%) are achieved when more than 200 consecutive cases of ESD have been performed [84]. This volume of experience is easily reached in Japan and East Asia but not in the West. Japanese and Western cr-ESD implementation protocols should be tailored on prognostics of difficulty, and quality outcomes for each gradient of difficulty should be standardized and used as key performance indicators. Given all data that are accumulating to support the safety and efficacy of ESD in the hands of skilled endoscopists, it is only a matter of time before it becomes more widely available outside of Asia. One of the major hurdles of disseminating ESD would be determining how and who should be certified to practice.

Conclusion

ESD is a reliable technique for achieving en bloc resection of large colorectal superficial neoplasms with superior curability and pathological evaluation compared to piecemeal EMR. Colorectal ESD reduces unnecessary surgery of mucosal carcinomas and improves the quality of life for patients with lower rectal lesions. Given its technical difficulties, colorectal ESD has specific indications, and the appropriate approach should be selected according to pretreatment tumor characterization. Further development of training systems will promote a worldwide standardization of the procedure. Ex vivo and in vivo animal training programs may provide the best chance to enhance safety and effectiveness of learning curves in Western countries. Developments of new devices and strategies resulted in improvements of outcomes. ESD adoption should continue to steadily increase in the coming years, and reimbursement guidelines based on key performance indicators will be required to guarantee the best outcomes.

Acknowledgments We would like to thank Dr. Shigeki Sekine and Hirokazu Taniguchi, Division of Pathology and Clinical Laboratory, National Cancer Center Hospital, Tokyo, Japan, and Dr. Patrizia Rigato, Pathology Unit Ospedale S. Giuseppe, Albano L, Rome, Italy, for providing clinicopathological suggestions.

We also would like to thank Dr. Takahisa Matsuda, Takeshi Nakajima, Taku Sakamoto, Seiichiro Abe, Masayoshi Yamada, Masau Sekiguchi, and Hiroyuki Takamaru, Endoscopy Division, National Cancer Center Hospital, Tokyo, Japan, for contributing to our ESD case series and data analysis. Finally, we would like to thank Dr. Agostino Scozzarro, former Chief of Digestive Endoscopy Unit for his hentusiastic support to organize an ESD Service in a Western Public Hospital; Dr. Narciso Mostarda, Hospital General Manager, for providing technical and amministrative support; and Prof. Guido Costamagna for his mentorship.

Disclosure This work was supported in part by the National Cancer Center Research and Development Fund (25-A-12 and 28-K-1) to Dr. Saito. The other authors disclosed no financial relationships relevant to this publication.

Competing Interests None.

References

1. Winawer SJ, Zauber AG, Ho MN, et al. Prevention of colorectal cancer by colonoscopic polypectomy. The national polyp study workgroup. N Engl J Med. 1993;329:1977–81.
2. Doubeni CA, Corley DA, Quinn VP, et al. Effectiveness of screening colonoscopy in reducing the risk of death from right and left colon cancer: a large community-based study. Gut. 2016.

3. Ahlenstiel G, Hourigan LF, Brown G, et al. Actual endoscopic versus predicted surgical mortality for treatment of advanced mucosal neoplasia of the colon. Gastrointest Endosc. 2014;80:668–76.
4. Tanaka S, Kashida H, Saito Y, et al. JGES guidelines for colorectal endoscopic submucosal dissection/endoscopic mucosal resection. Dig Endosc. 2015;27:417–34.
5. Pimentel-Nunes P, Dinis-Ribeiro M, Ponchon T, et al. Endoscopic submucosal dissection: European society of gastrointestinal endoscopy (ESGE) Guideline. Endoscopy. 2015;47:829–54.
6. Tanaka S, Oka S, Kaneko I, et al. Endoscopic submucosal dissection for colorectal neoplasia: possibility of standardization. Gastrointest Endosc. 2007;66:100–7.
7. Saito Y, Uraoka T, Yamaguchi Y, et al. A prospective, multicenter study of 1111 colorectal endoscopic submucosal dissections (with video). Gastrointest Endosc. 2010;72:1217–25.
8. Tanaka S, Tamegai Y, Tsuda S, et al. Multicenter questionnaire survey on the current situation of colorectal endoscopic submucosal dissection in Japan. Dig Endosc. 2010;22(Suppl 1):S2–8.
9. Saito Y, Fukuzawa M, Matsuda T, et al. Clinical outcome of endoscopic submucosal dissection versus endoscopic mucosal resection of large colorectal tumors as determined by curative resection. Surg Endosc. 2010;24:343–52.
10. Kobayashi N, Yoshitake N, Hirahara Y, et al. Matched case-control study comparing endoscopic submucosal dissection and endoscopic mucosal resection for colorectal tumors. J Gastroenterol Hepatol. 2012;27:728–33.
11. Puli SR, Kakugawa Y, Saito Y, et al. Successful complete cure en-bloc resection of large non-pedunculated colonic polyps by endoscopic submucosal dissection: a meta-analysis and systematic review. Ann Surg Oncol. 2009;16:2147–51.
12. Kwon CI. Endoscopic submucosal dissection (ESD) training and performing ESD with accurate and safe techniques. Clin Endosc. 2012;45:347–9.
13. Deprez PH, Bergman JJ, Meisner S, et al. Current practice with endoscopic submucosal dissection in Europe: position statement from a panel of experts. Endoscopy. 2010;42:853–8.
14. Tanaka S, Haruma K, Oka S, et al. Clinicopathologic features and endoscopic treatment of superficially spreading colorectal neoplasms larger than 20 mm. Gastrointest Endosc. 2001;54:62–6.
15. Kudo S. Endoscopic mucosal resection of flat and depressed types of early colorectal cancer. Endoscopy. 1993;25:455–61.
16. Uraoka T, Saito Y, Matsuda T, et al. Endoscopic indications for endoscopic mucosal resection of laterally spreading tumours in the colorectum. Gut. 2006;55:1592–7.
17. Oka S, Tanaka S, Kanao H, et al. Therapeutic strategy for colorectal laterally spreading tumor. Dig Endosc. 2009;21(Suppl 1):S43–6.
18. Moss A, Bourke MJ, Williams SJ, et al. Endoscopic mucosal resection outcomes and prediction of submucosal cancer from advanced colonic mucosal neoplasia. Gastroenterology. 2011;140:1909–18.
19. Kudo SE, Kashida H. Flat and depressed lesions of the colorectum. Clin Gastroenterol Hepatol. 2005;3:S33–6.
20. Kudo S, Lambert R, Allen JI, et al. Nonpolypoid neoplastic lesions of the colorectal mucosa. Gastrointest Endosc. 2008;68:S3–47.
21. The Paris endoscopic classification of superficial neoplastic lesions: esophagus, stomach, and colon: November 30 to December 1, 2002. Gastrointest Endosc. 2003;58:S3–43.
22. Kudo S, Tamura S, Nakajima T, et al. Diagnosis of colorectal tumorous lesions by magnifying endoscopy. Gastrointest Endosc. 1996;44:8–14.
23. Sano Y, Tanaka S, Kudo SE, et al. Narrow-band imaging (NBI) magnifying endoscopic classification of colorectal tumors proposed by the Japan NBI Expert Team. Dig Endosc. 2016(5):526–33.
24. Kanao H, Tanaka S, Oka S, et al. Clinical significance of type V(I) pit pattern subclassification in determining the depth of invasion of colorectal neoplasms. World J Gastroenterol. 2008;14:211–7.
25. Kobayashi Y, Kudo SE, Miyachi H, et al. Clinical usefulness of pit patterns for detecting colonic lesions requiring surgical treatment. Int J Color Dis. 2011;26:1531–40.

26. Buchner AM, Guarner-Argente C, Ginsberg GG. Outcomes of EMR of defiant colorectal lesions directed to an endoscopy referral center. Gastrointest Endosc. 2012;76:255–63.
27. Veerappan SG, Ormonde D, Yusoff IF, et al. Hot avulsion: a modification of an existing technique for management of nonlifting areas of a polyp (with video). Gastrointest Endosc. 2014;80:884–8.
28. Tsiamoulos ZP, Bourikas LA, Saunders BP. Endoscopic mucosal ablation: a new argon plasma coagulation/injection technique to assist complete resection of recurrent, fibrotic colon polyps (with video). Gastrointest Endosc. 2012;75:400–4.
29. Chedgy FJ, Bhattacharyya R, Kandiah K, et al. Knife-assisted snare resection: a novel technique for resection of scarred polyps in the colon. Endoscopy. 2016;48:277–80.
30. Sakamoto T, Saito Y, Matsuda T, et al. Treatment strategy for recurrent or residual colorectal tumors after endoscopic resection. Surg Endosc. 2011;25:255–60.
31. Rahmi G, Tanaka S, Ohara Y, et al. Efficacy of endoscopic submucosal dissection for residual or recurrent superficial colorectal tumors after endoscopic mucosal resection. J Dig Dis. 2015;16:14–21.
32. Kuroki Y, Hoteya S, Mitani T, et al. Endoscopic submucosal dissection for residual/locally recurrent lesions after endoscopic therapy for colorectal tumors. J Gastroenterol Hepatol. 2010;25:1747–53.
33. Rutter MD, Riddell RH. Colorectal dysplasia in inflammatory bowel disease: a clinicopathologic perspective. Clin Gastroenterol Hepatol. 2014;12:359–67.
34. Hurlstone DP, Sanders DS, Atkinson R, et al. Endoscopic mucosal resection for flat neoplasia in chronic ulcerative colitis: can we change the endoscopic management paradigm? Gut. 2007;56:838–46.
35. Iacopini F, Saito Y, Yamada M, et al. Curative endoscopic submucosal dissection of large nonpolypoid superficial neoplasms in ulcerative colitis (with videos). Gastrointest Endosc. 2015;82:734–8.
36. Higaki S, Hashimoto S, Harada K, et al. Long-term follow-up of large flat colorectal tumors resected endoscopically. Endoscopy. 2003;35:845–9.
37. Nakajima T, Saito Y, Tanaka S, et al. Current status of endoscopic resection strategy for large, early colorectal neoplasia in Japan. Surg Endosc. 2013;27:3262–70.
38. Oka S, Tanaka S, Saito Y, et al. Local recurrence after endoscopic resection for large colorectal neoplasia: a multicenter prospective study in Japan. Am J Gastroenterol. 2015;110:697–707.
39. Yamamoto S, Uedo N, Ishihara R, et al. Endoscopic submucosal dissection for early gastric cancer performed by supervised residents: assessment of feasibility and learning curve. Endoscopy. 2009;41:923–8.
40. Yamamoto Y, Fujisaki J, Ishiyama A, et al. Current status of training for endoscopic submucosal dissection for gastric epithelial neoplasm at cancer institute hospital, Japanese foundation for cancer research, a famous Japanese hospital. Dig Endosc. 2012;24(Suppl 1):148–53.
41. Draganov PV, Chang M, Coman RM, et al. Role of observation of live cases done by Japanese experts in the acquisition of ESD skills by a western endoscopist. World J Gastroenterol. 2014;20:4675–80.
42. Saito Y, Otake Y, Sakamoto T, et al. Indications for and technical aspects of colorectal endoscopic submucosal dissection. Gut Liver. 2013;7:263–9.
43. Kim EY, Jeon SW, Kim GH. Chicken soup for teaching and learning ESD. World J Gastroenterol. 2011;17:2618–22.
44. Gotoda T, Friedland S, Hamanaka H, et al. A learning curve for advanced endoscopic resection. Gastrointest Endosc. 2005;62:866–7.
45. Kakushima N, Fujishiro M, Kodashima S, et al. A learning curve for endoscopic submucosal dissection of gastric epithelial neoplasms. Endoscopy. 2006;38:991–5.
46. Oda I, Odagaki T, Suzuki H, et al. Learning curve for endoscopic submucosal dissection of early gastric cancer based on trainee experience. Dig Endosc. 2012;24(Suppl 1):129–32.
47. Tsuji Y, Ohata K, Sekiguchi M, et al. An effective training system for endoscopic submucosal dissection of gastric neoplasm. Endoscopy. 2011;43:1033–8.

48. Sakamoto T, Saito Y, Fukunaga S, et al. Learning curve associated with colorectal endoscopic submucosal dissection for endoscopists experienced in gastric endoscopic submucosal dissection. Dis Colon Rectum. 2011;54:1307–12.
49. Hotta K, Oyama T, Shinohara T, et al. Learning curve for endoscopic submucosal dissection of large colorectal tumors. Dig Endosc. 2010;22:302–6.
50. Probst A, Golger D, Anthuber M, et al. Endoscopic submucosal dissection in large sessile lesions of the rectosigmoid: learning curve in a European center. Endoscopy. 2012;44:660–7.
51. Niimi K, Goto O, Fujishiro M, et al. Endoscopic mucosal resection with a ligation device or endoscopic submucosal dissection for rectal carcinoid tumors: an analysis of 24 consecutive cases. Dig Endosc. 2012;24:443–7.
52. Shiga H, Endo K, Kuroha M, et al. Endoscopic submucosal dissection for colorectal neoplasia during the clinical learning curve. Surg Endosc. 2014;28:2120–8.
53. Suzuki H, Gotoda T, Sasako M, et al. Detection of early gastric cancer: misunderstanding the role of mass screening. Gastric Cancer. 2006;9:315–9.
54. Ribeiro-Mourao F, Pimentel-Nunes P, Dinis-Ribeiro M. Endoscopic submucosal dissection for gastric lesions: results of an European inquiry. Endoscopy. 2010;42:814–9.
55. Iacopini F, Bella A, Costamagna G, et al. Stepwise training in rectal and colonic endoscopic submucosal dissection with differentiated learning curves. Gastrointest Endosc. 2012;76:1188–96.
56. Yang DH, Jeong GH, Song Y, et al. The feasibility of performing colorectal endoscopic submucosal dissection without previous experience in performing gastric endoscopic submucosal dissection. Dig Dis Sci. 2015;60:3431–41.
57. Ohata K, Nonaka K, Misumi Y, et al. Usefulness of training using animal models for colorectal endoscopic submucosal dissection: is experience performing gastric ESD really needed? Endosc Int Open. 2016;4:E333–9.
58. Hon SS, Ng SS, Lee JF, et al. In vitro porcine training model for colonic endoscopic submucosal dissection: an inexpensive and safe way to acquire a complex endoscopic technique. Surg Endosc. 2010;24:2439–43.
59. Yoshida N, Yagi N, Inada Y, et al. Possibility of ex vivo animal training model for colorectal endoscopic submucosal dissection. Int J Color Dis. 2013;28:49–56.
60. Kato M, Gromski M, Jung Y, et al. The learning curve for endoscopic submucosal dissection in an established experimental setting. Surg Endosc. 2013;27:154–61.
61. Pioche M, Rivory J, Aguero-Garcete G, et al. New isolated bovine colon model dedicated to colonic ESD hands-on training: development and first evaluation. Surg Endosc. 2015;29:3209–15.
62. Rahmi G, Hotayt B, Chaussade S, et al. Endoscopic submucosal dissection for superficial rectal tumors: prospective evaluation in France. Endoscopy. 2014;46:670–6.
63. Moss A, Bourke MJ, Tran K, et al. Lesion isolation by circumferential submucosal incision prior to endoscopic mucosal resection (CSI-EMR) substantially improves en bloc resection rates for 40-mm colonic lesions. Endoscopy. 2010;42:400–4.
64. Sakamoto T, Matsuda T, Nakajima T, et al. Efficacy of endoscopic mucosal resection with circumferential incision for patients with large colorectal tumors. Clin Gastroenterol Hepatol. 2012;10:22–6.
65. Terasaki M, Tanaka S, Oka S, et al. Clinical outcomes of endoscopic submucosal dissection and endoscopic mucosal resection for laterally spreading tumors larger than 20 mm. J Gastroenterol Hepatol. 2012;27:734–40.
66. Sakamoto T, Matsuda T, Otake Y, et al. Predictive factors of local recurrence after endoscopic piecemeal mucosal resection. J Gastroenterol. 2012;47:635–40.
67. Toyonaga T, Man IM, Morita Y, et al. The new resources of treatment for early stage colorectal tumors: EMR with small incision and simplified endoscopic submucosal dissection. Dig Endosc. 2009;21(Suppl 1):S31–7.
68. Kim YJ, Kim ES, Cho KB, et al. Comparison of clinical outcomes among different endoscopic resection methods for treating colorectal neoplasia. Dig Dis Sci. 2013;58:1727–36.

69. Fujishiro M, Yahagi N, Kashimura K, et al. Comparison of various submucosal injection solutions for maintaining mucosal elevation during endoscopic mucosal resection. Endoscopy. 2004;36:579–83.

70. Ciocirlan M, Pioche M, Lepilliez V, et al. The ENKI-2 water-jet system versus dual knife for endoscopic submucosal dissection of colorectal lesions: a randomized comparative animal study. Endoscopy. 2014;46:139–43.

71. Takeuchi Y, Shimokawa T, Ishihara R, et al. An electrosurgical endoknife with a water-jet function (flushknife) proves its merits in colorectal endoscopic submucosal dissection especially for the cases which should be removed en bloc. Gastroenterol Res Pract. 2013;2013:530123.

72. Harada A, Gotoda T, Fukuzawa M, et al. Clinical impact of endoscopic devices for colorectal endoscopic submucosal dissection. Digestion. 2013;88:72–8.

73. Jacques J, Kerever S, Carrier P, et al. HybridKnife high-pressure glycerol jet injection for endoscopic submucosal dissection increases procedural ease and speed: a randomised study in pigs and a human case series. Surg Endosc. 2016;30:3152–9.

74. Sakamoto H, Hayashi Y, Miura Y, et al. Pocket-creation method facilitates endoscopic submucosal dissection of colorectal laterally spreading tumors, non-granular type. Endosc Int Open. 2017;5:E123–9.

75. Oyama T. Counter traction makes endoscopic submucosal dissection easier. Clin Endosc. 2012;45:375–8.

76. Ritsuno H, Sakamoto N, Osada T, et al. Prospective clinical trial of traction device-assisted endoscopic submucosal dissection of large superficial colorectal tumors using the S-O clip. Surg Endosc. 2014;28:3143–9.

77. Hori K, Uraoka T, Harada K, et al. Predictive factors for technically difficult endoscopic submucosal dissection in the colorectum. Endoscopy. 2014;46:862–70.

78. Imai K, Hotta K, Yamaguchi Y, et al. Preoperative indicators of failure of en bloc resection or perforation in colorectal endoscopic submucosal dissection: implications for lesion stratification by technical difficulties during stepwise training. Gastrointest Endosc. 2016;83:954–62.

79. Isomoto H, Nishiyama H, Yamaguchi N, et al. Clinicopathological factors associated with clinical outcomes of endoscopic submucosal dissection for colorectal epithelial neoplasms. Endoscopy. 2009;41:679–83.

80. Mizushima T, Kato M, Iwanaga I, et al. Technical difficulty according to location, and risk factors for perforation, in endoscopic submucosal dissection of colorectal tumors. Surg Endosc. 2015;29:133–9.

81. Sato K, Ito S, Kitagawa T, et al. Factors affecting the technical difficulty and clinical outcome of endoscopic submucosal dissection for colorectal tumors. Surg Endosc. 2014;28:2959–65.

82. Takeuchi Y, Iishi H, Tanaka S, et al. Factors associated with technical difficulties and adverse events of colorectal endoscopic submucosal dissection: retrospective exploratory factor analysis of a multicenter prospective cohort. Int J Color Dis. 2014;29:1275–84.

83. Hayashi N, Tanaka S, Nishiyama S, et al. Predictors of incomplete resection and perforation associated with endoscopic submucosal dissection for colorectal tumors. Gastrointest Endosc. 2014;79:427–35.

84. Tanaka S, Terasaki M, Hayashi N, et al. Warning for unprincipled colorectal endoscopic submucosal dissection: accurate diagnosis and reasonable treatment strategy. Dig Endosc. 2013;25:107–16.

Submucosal Injection Solutions for Colon Polypectomy

7

Antonio Facciorusso and Nicola Muscatiello

7.1   Introduction

As widely described in previous chapters of this book, colon polypectomy either through endoscopic mucosal resection (EMR) and endoscopic submucosal dissection (ESD) is a standard procedure for treating noninvasive mucosal adenomas and neoplasms, with the aim to interrupt the adenoma-carcinoma sequence leading to invasive cancer [1, 2]. EMR and ESD are usually performed through the injection of a fluid agent into the submucosal space to expand it, rendering polypectomy easier and safer ("inject-and-cut" technique) [3, 4]. In particular, bleeding is the most frequent adverse event of endoscopic polypectomy, especially in the case of large pedunculated or flat lesions, with a reported incidence ranging from 0.3 to 6.1% and can occur up to 3 weeks after the procedure [4].

Several injection solutions have been tested and are currently used to create a submucosal cushion delimiting the lesion from the muscularis propria, so allowing the complete resection of the lesion and preventing perforation and thermal injury to the gastrointestinal (GI) wall.

Normal saline (NS) solution is most commonly used in clinical practice because of its low cost and ease of use. However, NS often requires repeated injections because of its rapid absorption into the surrounding tissue, thus increasing the risk of piecemeal resection and theoretically hampering the overall efficacy of the procedure [5].

This aspect pushed the endoscopy community to test various submucosal injection solutions such as hyaluronic acid (HA), glycerol, dextrose water (DW), fibrinogen mixture (FM), polidocanol, and hydroxypropyl methylcellulose (HPMC) in order to fulfill the pressing need of the ideal agent for EMR and ESD [6].

A. Facciorusso (✉) • N. Muscatiello
Gastroenterology Unit, Department of Medical Sciences, University of Foggia,
AOU Ospedali Riuniti, Viale Pinto, 1, 71100 Foggia, Italy
e-mail: antonio.facciorusso@virgilio.it

© Springer International Publishing AG 2018
A. Facciorusso, N. Muscatiello (eds.), *Colon Polypectomy*,
https://doi.org/10.1007/978-3-319-59457-6_7

89

Such substances have been tested due to their ability to create a longer-lasting submucosal cushion as a result of their viscous properties. In doing so, they should be potentially able to allow lengthier procedures and increase the rate of en bloc resection, even for large lesions [7, 8].

However, despite the promising results of the preliminary reports, their efficacy in preventing the main complication after polypectomy, namely, postpolypectomy bleeding (PPB), is still a matter of debate.

An ideal submucosal injection solution should be inexpensive, readily available, nontoxic, and easy to prepare and inject and should provide a long-lasting submucosal cushion [9]. It should also provide a sufficiently high submucosal elevation to facilitate an en bloc resection (to reduce the local recurrence rate) and reduce the risk of perforation [10].

Unfortunately, none of the aforementioned substances seem to fulfill all these features.

Table 7.1 summarizes the characteristics of the various submucosal injection solutions tested so far.

Table 7.1 Submucosal injection solutions for EMR and ESD

Solution	Submucosal lift duration	Cost	Advantages	Disadvantages
Normal saline	+	+	Cheap, readily available, easy to inject, safe	Rapidly re-adsorbed
Hypertonic saline	++	+	Cheap, readily available, easy to inject	Local complications such as inflammation and tissue damage
Hyaluronic acid	+++	+++	Determines the longest-lasting cushion, high en bloc rate, low risk of perforation	Expensive, not widely available, very viscous, seems to stimulate the proliferation of residual adenoma cells
Glycerol	++	+	Cheap, readily available	Smoke production
Dextrose	++	+	Cheap, readily available	Local inflammation, tissue damage
Fibrinogen mixture	+++	++	Long-lasting cushion, easy to use, microvascular hemostatic effect which helps to keep the field clean, not expensive	Limited availability, risk of contamination/infection spread
Hydroxypropyl methylcellulose	+++	++	Long-lasting cushion, not expensive	Local inflammation, tissue damage, high viscosity

Table 7.1 (continued)

Solution	Submucosal lift duration	Cost	Advantages	Disadvantages
Succinylated gelatin	+++	+	Cheap, long-lasting cushion, easy to use, readily available	Limited data, no apparent benefit in preventing bleeding
Autologous blood	+++	++	Long-lasting cushion, not expensive	Limited data, risk of clotting in syringe
Polidocanol	+++	+	Long-lasting cushion, not expensive, lower risk of bleeding due to its sclerosing activity	Theoretical risk of wall necrosis and perforation, need to confirmation in randomized trials

EMR endoscopic mucosal resection, *ESD* endoscopic submucosal dissection

Since the appropriate selection of submucosal injection solutions is important for successful EMR and ESD, in this review we aim to address recent advances in this field. Physical characteristics of various submucosal injection solutions are also described.

7.2 Submucosal Injection Solutions

7.2.1 Normal Saline Solution

Normal saline has been one of the first solutions to be adopted in colon polypectomy due to its low cost, safety, and ease of use. Therefore, NS is still currently the most used solution for EMR worldwide and the agent for which most literature is available. However, the greatest issue with NS is the rapid dissipation of the submucosal cushion which often requires more injections thus increasing the risk of piecemeal resection [6, 11]. This may represent a real problem particularly for flat elevated lesions or large lesions for which maintaining a long-lasting submucosal cushion at a proper height is of paramount importance. Noteworthy, flat and large pedunculated polyps are specifically those at higher need of fluid solution injection, while use of "injection-and-cut" technique for small and non-flat lesions is more questionable.

These findings have been confirmed in a recent meta-analysis of five RCTs which found NS significantly inferior to viscous hypertonic solutions (hydroxyethyl starch, 50% dextrose, sodium hyaluronate, succinylated gelatin, and hyaluronic acid) in terms of en bloc resection rate of lesions >2 cm [Odds ratio (OR): 2.09, 1.15–3.80; $p = 0.02$], while a slighter difference was registered for smaller polyps (OR: 1.21, 0.32–4.60; $p = 0.78$) [12].

Dilute epinephrine (1:100,000–1:200,000) is often added to NS fluid due to the theoretical benefits of decreased bleeding and a sustained submucosal cushion (due to delayed absorption of fluid resulting from decreased vascular flow and vasoconstriction) with no apparent increase in side effects [13]. Only anecdotal case reports on systemic catecholaminergic effects (hypertension, tachycardia, ischemia) have been published, and serious concerns on NS + epinephrine injection can be excluded [14–16].

In spite of the promising results of a preliminary retrospective study [17], two prospective randomized controlled trials (RCTs) failed to report a significant advantage of submucosal injection of dilute epinephrine as compared to NS alone in preventing delayed PPB [18, 19]. Only Hsieh's study found a slight benefit of epinephrine over NS as for immediate bleeding [18], but delayed PPB (well-known to be usually more severe) rate did not differ between the two groups.

In a recent meta-analysis of seven RCTs, epinephrine injection determined a pooled risk ratio (RR) 0.37 (95% confidence interval 0.20–0.66; $p = 0.001$) when compared to no prophylaxis, while it resulted inferior to other mechanical procedures such as loop or clips [20]. Of note, a network meta-analysis published this year confirmed epinephrine-saline injection as effective in preventing early PPB (RR: 0.32, 0.11–0.67) but failed to find any prophylactic measure (epinephrine-NS injection, mechanical therapy, or combined) as associated to lower delayed PPB [21].

Table 7.2 reports the main characteristics of RCTs comparing epinephrine-saline injection to other/no prophylactic measures for PPB [18, 19, 22–26].

Staining dye (i.e., diluted indigo carmine or methylene blue) is frequently added to the injection solution to facilitate identification of the margins of the target lesion before and during resection [27]. Staining dye may also help in early identifying tissue injury and perforation [27].

7.2.2 Hypertonic Saline Solution

Hypertonic saline (HS) solution shares a number of advantages of NS, namely, it is inexpensive, readily available, and easy-to-inject but creates a higher submucosal cushion than normal saline [6, 28].

However, some concerns have been raised on a non-negligible risk of tissue damage and local inflammation after hypertonic sodium chloride injection due to its higher osmolarity [29]. Animal studies comparing several different submucosal injection solutions found considerable tissue damage with 3.75% NaCl and dextrose water (DW) injection visualized mainly as mucosal erosion which persisted a week after the procedure [29]. Histological specimen examination showed degradation of epithelial glands, congestion of capillary vessels, and finally fibrosis of submucosal layer a week after injection [29].

Due to the aforementioned drawbacks, HS is not used routinely in the clinical practice.

Table 7.2 Randomized controlled trials comparing epinephrine-saline injection with other/no prophylactic therapy for postpolypectomy bleeding

Study, year	Country	Period	Treatment	Polyp size (mm)	Early bleeding	Delayed bleeding
Rohde, 2000 [22]	Germany	NR	A: Epinephrine-NS (20) B: None (20)	A: 15 (7–28) B: 15 (11–35)	A: 1 (5%) B: 5 (25%)	A: 0 (0%) B: 0 (0%)
Hsieh, 2001 [18]	Taiwan	1997–1999	A: Epinephrine-NS (39) B: None (48)	NA	A: 0 (0%) B: 2 (4.2%)	A: 0 (0%) B: 0 (0%)
Di Giorgio, 2004 [23]	Italy	1995–2002	A: Detachable snare (163) B: Epinephrine-NS (161) C: None (164)	A: 22.2 ± 5.9 B: 24.7 ± 5.3 C: 21.6 ± 4.8	A: 2 (1.2%) B: 3 (1.9%) C: 10 (6.1%)	A: 1 (0.6%) B: 2 (1.2%) C: 3 (1.8%)
Dobrowolski, 2004 [24]	Poland	2000–2002	A: Epinephrine-NS (50) B: None (50)	A: 16.3 ± 5.4 B: 16.1 ± 5.9	A: 1 (2%) B: 8 (16%)	A: 0 (0%) B: 0 (0%)
Paspatis, 2006 [25]	Greece	NR	A: Snare + Epinephrine-NS (84) B: Epinephrine-NS (75)	A: 27.1 ± 8.9 B: 26.3 ± 8.1	A: 1 (1.2%) B: 7 (9.3%)	A: 1 (1.2%) B: 1 (1.3%)
Kouklakis 2009 [26]	Greece	2004–2007	A: Endoloop with clipping (32) B: Epinephrine-NS (32)	A: 25.6 ± 12 B: 27 ± 11	A: 0 (0%) B: 2 (6.3%)	A: 1 (3.1%) B: 2 (6.3%)

NR not reported, *NS* normal saline

7.2.3 Glycerol

A more promising hypertonic agent is glycerol solution consisting of 10% glycerin and 5% fructose in a NS solution. Glycerol is safely used intravenously as an osmotic agent against cerebral edema, [30] and it has been used in interventional endoscopy since the first report in 1995 [31].

Since then, a few studies have evaluated its effect as a submucosal injection solution.

In an in vitro study comparing glycerol and NS conducted on fresh resected human colon specimens, glycerol group maintained significantly longer-lasting submucosal elevation, and the hemispheric shape produced by glycerol solution facilitated snaring satisfactorily [32].

Based on this finding, Uraoka et al. retrospectively compared the en bloc and complete resection rates as well as safety of EMR of colorectal laterally spreading tumors (LSTs) performed either through glycerol or NS injection [33]. En bloc resection rate was 63.6% (70/110) in the glycerol group and 48.9% (55/113) in the

NS group ($p = 0.03$). Subgroup analysis based on lesion size confirmed superiority of glycerol solution in LSTs <20 mm ($p < 0.01$) but found no significant difference in greater lesions (≥20 mm) [33]. Therefore, although glycerol provides higher overall en bloc resection rates, it does not seem to increase the efficacy of EMR in those lesions more difficult to remove.

The rate of associated complications such as perforations and delayed PPB was similar in both groups [33]. These results led to a wide use of glycerol as injection solution for EMR in a number of countries such as Japan [11].

As reported in the above-cited animal study and confirmed in vivo by Uraoka et al., glycerol does not determine any apparent mucosal damage nor histological tissue alteration [29, 33]. In the discussion to their study, Fujishiro et al. acknowledge the favorable cost-effectiveness of glycerol which, although appears slightly inferior to hyaluronic acid (HA) as to safety and lesion-lifting ability, is considerably cheaper [29]. Authors speculate that the excellent safety of glycerol is mainly due to its ability to pass freely through the cell membrane, because the osmotic pressure difference between the inside and the outside of the cell membrane is only generated by an additional use of 5% fructose in the solution, which causes no cell destruction [33]. On the contrary, because osmotic pressure of glycerol is approximately seven times higher than the extracellular fluid, glycerol is able to produce sufficient submucosal cushion [33].

In conclusion, glycerol appears as a very promising agent for colon EMR but needs further confirmation in RCTs as all clinical reports are currently only from small Eastern retrospective series.

7.2.4   Dextrose Water

Among the most frequently used hypertonic solutions, properties of dextrose water (DW) have been extensively described. DW presents many of the features of an ideal injection solution: it produces and maintains high and long-lasting mucosal elevation, it is cheap, widely available, and easy to inject [34, 35]. Varadarajulu et al. found 50% DW superior to NS in terms of en bloc resection rate (82% vs 44%; $p = 0.01$) with need of smaller volumes (median 7 mL vs 5 mL; $p = 0.02$) and fewer injections (median 2 vs 1; $p = 0.003$) and similar complication rate [34]. Similar efficacy results were found by Katsinelos et al. who compared 50% DW plus epinephrine versus NS plus epinephrine during EMRs of sessile rectosigmoid polyps (>10 mm) [36]. However, despite the findings of Varadarajulu's report, this study raised concerns about the safety of DW solution since the risk of thermal tissue injury (e.g., postpolypectomy syndrome) was significantly higher than in the NS plus epinephrine group [36].

The aforementioned animal study comparing several injection solutions tested the mucosal effects of DW at five different concentrations (5, 10, 15, 30, and 40%) and registered considerable tissue damage with DW at concentrations ≥20% with milder alterations (mucosal whiteness with marginal redness lasting less than a week) observed even with 15% DW [29]. DW at 20% produced tissue changes similar to those observed with hypertonic saline solution (see above), while in 30, 40, and 50% DW, shallow ulcerations were formed a day after injection and persisted a week after injection [29]. Of note, histological examination showed not only mucosal damage but even muscle layer damage in 30, 40, and 50% DW-injected pigs [29].

The most studied DW solution in clinical trials is 50% DW, which was tested in three RCTs [34, 35, 37] of which two comparing 50% DW to NS [33, 34] and one to sodium hyaluronate (SH) [37]. A recent systematic review and meta-analysis found only nonsignificant trends in favor of 50% DW both in terms of complete resection rate [odds ratio (OR): 1.12 (0.69–1.80) vs NS and 1.04 (0.65–1.68) vs SH] and bleeding rate (OR: 0.54, 0.11–2.57 vs NS and 0.25, 0.03–2.26 vs SH) with considerably higher complication rate [38].

Based on these findings, use of DW at a concentration $\geq 15\%$ is highly discouraged due to the high risk of mucosal ulcers and damage of the resected specimen with consequent inaccurate histopathological assessment [39].

7.2.5 Hyaluronic Acid

Hyaluronic acid (HA) is a type of glycosaminoglycan found in connective tissue, commonly used for intra-articular injections in osteoarthritis patients and in eye surgery [40, 41].

The efficacy of HA in EMR has been previously tested in animal models [28, 42–44].

Yoshida et al. compared in a porcine model 0.9% NS and four concentrations of 800-kDa HA (0.4, 0.2, 0.13, and 0.1%) [42]. All concentrations of HA solution maintained greater mucosal elevation at all times than NS ($p < 0.05$), and mucosal elevation diminished 2 min after the submucosal injection with NS but was maintained 2 min after injection with 0.4, 0.2, and 0.13% HA [42].

Similar results were found by Hyun et al. who demonstrated that the mucosal elevation induced by 0.1% HA lasted longer than the elevation by NS or by mannitol in a resected mongrel colon [43].

In the previously cited animal study by Fujishiro et al., two solutions of HA (0.25% 1900 kDa and 0.125% 1900 kDa) were found to be safe and not to determine any significant tissue damage after injection [29]. Therefore, authors concluded that HA solution may be the best with regard to tissue damage as well as to its lesion-lifting ability because it is a thick substance with high viscoelasticity and it is not antigenic or toxic to humans, but its crucial disadvantage may be the high cost [29].

Based on these premises, HA has been tested in several clinical reports [45–50].

Yamamoto et al. found sodium hyaluronate safe and effective for en bloc resection of gastric lesions up to 20 mm [45] and large colonic tumors [46]. The same group conducted an open-label prospective study with 0.4% sodium hyaluronate in 40 patients with colon lesions up to 20 mm, finding an en bloc resection rate of 82.5% (33/40) and complication rate 10% (4/40) [47].

Moreover, HA resulted in a greater number of successful en bloc resections and lower perforation rates also in gastric and colorectal ESD [48–50].

Commercially available sodium hyaluronate solutions are usually too thick to inject through catheters and need dilution with NS before use, which increases the risk of contamination. In order to obviate to this issue, Kim et al. have recently evaluated a ready-to-use 0.4% sodium hyaluronate (Endo-Ease®, UNIMED Pharm. Inc., Seoul, Korea) in a multicenter RCT with 152 patients (72 with a gastric neoplasm and 82 with a colorectal neoplasm) [51]. The usefulness rate was significantly higher in the sodium hyaluronate group than in the NS group (89.2% vs 60.0% for gastric neoplasms and 95.3% vs 67.7% for colorectal neoplasms, $p < 0.001$) as well as ease of mucosal resection as perceived by the endoscopist ($p < 0.001$) [51]. The injected volume was even smaller than in the NS group ($p < 0.05$) [51].

Some authors raised concerns on the potential stimulation of the growth of residual tumor cells mainly due to increased CD44 expression of cancer cells at the wound sites induced by HA [52]. Therefore, HA should not be used for endoscopic piecemeal resection procedures because it increases the risk of residual tumors, while it appears to be an adequate agent for ESD [6].

Unfortunately, despite the optimal results in animal and clinical trials, the use of HA solutions in clinical practice is still limited by the costs.

Fujishiro et al. evaluated the possibility of developing an appropriate low-cost HA solution by diversifying its molecular weight and mixing it with various solutions such as glycerol or DW. They report that a mixture of 0.125% 1900 kDa sodium hyaluronate with 20% DW created a similar viscoelasticity to that of the 0.5% 800 kDa sodium hyauronate/NS solution [53]. Furthermore, the 0.125% 1900 kDa SH/glycerol solution created similar submucosal fluid cushions with a synergistic effect of increased viscoelasticity and the hypertonic nature of glycerin [53]. Therefore, authors concluded that a mixture of higher molecular weight sodium hyaluronate with a sugar solution (particularly 20% dextrose), with or without glycerin, should be regarded as a cost-effective option for colon polypectomy [53].

The same authors successfully tested the mixture of 1900 kDa HA (Suvenyl) with a 10% glycerin plus 5% fructose solution (Glyceol) in ESD of 67 large GI tumors in 54 patients [54]. Perforation occurred only once (1.5%) and was managed conservatively by endoscopic clipping, while endoscopic hemostasis was necessary twice (3%) because of postoperative bleeding [54]. Overall endoscopic and histologic en bloc resection rates were 94% (63/67) and 78% (52/67), respectively, and there was no recurrence after follow-up of 1 year [54].

A Western group published a series of 30 patients with 32 colonic and 1 duodenal lesions treated with an over-the-counter 0.15% HA preparation, which resulted safe, effective, and above all considerably cheaper than usual HA solutions [55]. Specifically, en bloc resection was achieved in 26 of the 28 lesions up to 25 mm in diameter, whereas all the lesions measuring 30–60 mm (5/32) required piecemeal resection; there was only one complication, a case of postpolypectomy bleeding [55].

In conclusion, HA has all the hallmarks of the ideal solution, but the high costs limited its use in clinical practice. Less expensive mixtures of HA at lower concentrations with other solutions need further confirmation.

7.2.6   Fibrinogen Mixture

Fibrinogen mixture (FM) entered clinical practice in 2004, when Lee et al. published a series of 35 early stage gastric neoplasms treated with EMR through FM injection [56]. Authors registered 82.9% en bloc resection rate and 88.6% complete resection rate, as a consequence of the properties of FM, namely, viscosity (which produces a long-lasting submucosal elevation that allows EMR without the need of additional injections), and the microvascular hemostatic effect (thereby keeping the visual field clear) [56]. These results were confirmed in a subsequent RCT comparing FM with NS solution in 72 patients with early gastric cancer (EGC) receiving EMR [57]. No significant differences were observed between the two groups (FM vs NS) in the rates of en bloc resection (80.6% vs 88.9%), complete resection rate (86.1% vs 80.6%), and recurrence rate (3% vs 6.1%), while mean procedure time was significantly shorter in the FM group (11.39 ± 3.07 min vs 13.93 ± 3.26 min; $p < 0.05$) [57]. Moreover, mean submucosal injection volume of the FM group was significantly lower (9.81 ± 2.26 mL vs 14.32 ± 2.35 mL; $p < 0.05$), and additional submucosal injections were less frequently required (5.6% vs 33.3%; $p < 0.05$) [57].

Therefore, FM may be a suitable submucosal injection solution and may be a good and cheaper alternative to HA [39], but being produced using coagulation proteins of human serum, it has the risk of transmitting hepatitis or other viruses due to the contamination of sera [11].

These safety concerns and the costs (less then HA but higher than NS) have limited the use of FM so far.

7.2.7   Hydroxypropyl Methylcellulose

Hydroxypropyl methylcellulose (HPMC) is a cellulose derivative with viscoelastic properties, primarily used by ophthalmologists in Western countries for creating artificial tears [58].

In a preliminary study, HPMC was found to create a long-lasting submucosal fluid cushion with minimal tissue damage [59]. Later animal studies confirmed the efficacy of HPMC for EMR of large mucosal lesions [43, 60, 61]; of note, duration of mucosal elevation was correlated with viscosity but not with osmolarity [43].

As already seen with HA, HPMC is very viscous and needs to be diluted before injection. Although HPMC is less expensive than HA, it is a synthetic product that may give rise to antigenic reactions (unlike HA), and robust data from clinical studies is still lacking [6]. Therefore, clear assumptions on HPMC routinely use cannot be drawn.

7.2.8   Succinylated Gelatin

Succinylated gelatin (SG) is a clear, inexpensive, 4% colloidal solution commonly available for intravenous resuscitation. Its pharmacological basis is that succinylation negatively charges the gelatin molecule resulting in spatial expansion, thereby occupying significantly more volume than non-succinylated protein chains of the same molecular weight [62]. As a consequence, when used intravenously, it has a long-lasting volume replacement effect, and its oncotic action is comparable with that of human albumin [62]. Moreover, SG has a favorable safety profile, and its only contraindication is history of gelatin hypersensitivity.

An animal study by Moss et al. found SG safe and determining a 42% increase in surface area for en bloc EMR as compared to NS [62]. Moreover, the median submucosal cushion duration was 60 min with SG versus 15 min with NS ($p < 0.005$), and median procedure duration with SG was 2.6 min vs 2.5 min with NS ($p = 0.515$) [62].

Based on these striking results, the same group conducted an RCT enrolling 80 patients with large colorectal sessile polyps ($\geq$ 20 mm) randomized either to SG (41 subjects) or NS (39 patients) [63].

The two groups did not differ as to complete single-session lesion excision rate (90% both) and safety profile, while a significant difference in favor of SG was found with regard to the primary endpoint, namely, a specific numeric parameter called "Sydney resection quotient" defined as lesion size in mm divided by the number of pieces to resect [63]. The median of this quotient was 10.0 (interquartile range, 7.5–20) in SG group and 5.9 (4.4–11.7) in NS patients ($p = 0.004$) [63]. Furthermore, SG resulted in fewer resections per lesion (3.0, 1.0–6.0 vs 5.5, 3.0–10.0 of NS; $p = 0.028$), fewer injections per lesion (2.0, 1.0–3.0 vs 3.0, 2.0–11.0; $p = 0.002$), lower injection volume (14.5 mL, 8.5–23.0 vs 20.0 mL, 16.0–46.0 with NS, $p = 0.009$), and shorter procedure duration (12.0 min, 8.0–28.0 vs 24.5 min, 15.0–36.0 with NS, $p = 0.006$) [63]. However, although authors concluded that SG almost halves the number of resections for piecemeal EMR as well as the procedure duration, PPB did not differ significantly between the two groups thus speaking in favor of a non-superiority of SG as for this important outcome [63].

Further clinical studies are warranted to confirm the promising results of SG.

7.2.9   Polidocanol

Polidocanol has been known as a sclerosing agent for several years and is broadly used in the treatment of esophageal varices, hemangiomas, and hemorrhoids. Following previous observations that at 1% concentration polidocanol presents a pro-coagulative effect with no risk of necrosis of deeper mucosa layers [64], our group decided to evaluate the efficacy of polidocanol injection in preventing PPB as compared to epinephrine solution in a series of 612 patients with large ($\geq$20 mm) LSTs or sessile polyps [65]. After propensity score matching, polidocanol resulted more effective in preventing both immediate and delayed PPB (3.9% vs 10.7% of control group, $p = 0.001$ and 1.3% vs 6.2% of control group, $p = 0.002$, respectively), and its efficacy was confirmed in almost all the subgroups regardless of polyp size and histology [65]. Severe complications were rare, and the two groups did not differ in number of snare resections for lesion and procedure duration ($p = 0.24$ and 0.6, respectively) [65].

In their editorial to our study, Repici et al. raised some concerns on the safety of polidocanol [66]; however, it should be noted that the theoretical harmful effects in promoting inflammation and mucosal necrosis, which have limited its use in polypectomy procedures so far, occurred only with concentrations superior to 2% and higher volumes since the extension of the damage is tightly dependent on the concentration and on the volume injected [65, 67].

On the contrary, since polidocanol solution contains ethanol, its electrical conductivity is significantly lower than saline solutions, and consequently the spread of thermal damage over mucosal layers is more limited [64].

Based on our promising results and the apparently favorable cost-effectiveness and safety profile, we consider polidocanol a valuable option for colon EMR which needs further confirmation in RCTs.

7.2.10 Autologous Blood

Encouraging results have been recently reported on the use of autologous blood for submucosal injection [8, 68, 69].

In a pivotal animal study comparing six solutions as cushioning agents in live pigs, animal's own whole blood resulted in significantly longer mucosal elevations than any other solution (namely, NS, NS plus epinephrine, albumin 12.5%, albumin 25%, and HPMC) [68].

Similar findings were obtained in another animal study conducted in a resected porcine stomach, where autologous blood resulted in considerably longer mucosal lifting and generated adequate mucosal elevation for the resection of high-quality specimens [69].

On the basis of these premises, a clinical Japanese study successfully performed EMR through submucosal injection of autologous blood in 28 patients with 35 colorectal polyps, with no increase in complications and obtaining optimal specimens for pathologic examination [70].

The specific properties of autologous blood offer several advantages: first, its corpuscular components allow prolonged submucosal elevation, while its procoagulatory mediators promote local hemostasis thus preventing PPB; second, it is inexpensive, readily available, and safe [6].

However, procoagulatory constituents in blood can cause clotting in the syringe if an injection is delayed, and further human data is needed to clarify the real role of autologous blood in the armamentarium for EMR and ESD.

7.2.11 Other Solutions

In addition to the above commented solutions, several other submucosal injection agents have been developed and experimented for EMR or ESD.

Carboxymethylcellulose (CMC) is commonly used as a viscosity modifier or thickener. Since it is reported to be nontoxic and nonallergenic [71], CMC has been considered a suitable injection agent to EMR. Burns et al. demonstrated in vitro that due to its high viscosity, CMC at concentrations greater than 2% was able to dissect the submucosal from the muscular layer [72].

Subsequently, Lenz et al. found CMC superior to NS and comparable to HPMC in terms of submucosal lifting duration (31 min vs 37 min for HPMC and only 19 for NS) in the stomach of nine pigs [61]. In another animal study, Yamasaki et al. compared various concentrations (0.5–3.5%) of CMC and confirmed that CMC solution dissects most of the mucosal layer from the muscular layer at the concentration above 2.0% [73]. Therefore, authors proposed 2.5% CMC as ideal submucosal agent for gastric ESD, as confirmed also in histopathological examinations which revealed no tissue damage [73]. Some concerns were raised on the high viscosity of the solution which required a special 18G submucosal injection needle catheter to minimize injection resistance in the aforementioned animal study [73]. By the way, no general indications on the use of CMC for EMR/ESD can be currently suggested given the lack of clinical studies.

Chitosan hydrogen (CH), a natural polysaccharide produced through deacetylation of chitotin, is a well-known viscous solution with hemostatic, anti-bacterial, and wound healing properties [74, 75].

Ishizuka et al. showed in an animal study with rat models that submucosal injection of CH produces a significantly thicker submucosal layer and reduced delayed bleeding as compared to hypertonic saline and HA [76]. Such results were confirmed by the same group in another animal study conducted on 18 pigs [77]. CH injection led to a longer-lasting elevation with clearer margins, compared with hypertonic saline, thus enabling precise ESD along the margins of the elevated mucosa; moreover, the endoscopic appearance after ESD was similar in both groups [77]. Finally, CH biodegradation was completed within 8 weeks according to endoscopic and histologic analyses [77].

Unfortunately, there is not yet enough reported evidence on the effectiveness and safety of CH in humans, so further clinical studies are warranted prior to actual clinical use.

Biodegradable hydrogels can deliver therapeutic payloads with great potentials in EMR and ESD to yield improvements in efficacy and foster mucosal regeneration.

Tran et al. compared an injectable drug-eluting elastomeric polymer (iDEEP) with NS and sodium hyaluronate in ex vivo porcine stomachs [78]. All EMR procedures were successfully performed after injection of iDEEP, and the elevation height of iDEEP (5.7 ± 0.5 mm) was higher than that of saline solution (2.8 ± 0.2 mm, $p < 0.01$) and sodium hyaluronate (4.2 ± 0.2 mm, $p < 0.05$) [78].

Sodium alginate was proved as effective as sodium hyaluronate as injection solution for EMR in an animal study with six dogs [79]. Histological examination of EMR-induced artificial ulcers revealed no apparent tissue damage and showed normal healing process, as confirmed in other series [79, 80]. These findings were confirmed in a small series of 11 patients undergoing gastric ESD [81]. In particular, ESD using sodium alginate was completed successfully in all patients without adverse effects except in one patient in whom transient shrinkage of the gastric wall disappeared spontaneously after approximately 30 min [81].

Interesting results were provided by an RCT comparing hydroxyethyl starch + epinephrine and NS + epinephrine in patients with colorectal LSTs ≥30 mm [82]. HES + E injection produced a more prolonged submucosal elevation (median 20.15 min; range, 9.6–13.4 vs 18.5 min, 14.5–28.4 in NS + epinephrine group; $p < 0.001$) and lowered overall procedure time (20.15 min, 12–32.5 vs 22.8 min, 18–34.5 in NS + epinephrine group); however, the safety of EMR was not influenced [82].

Table 7.3 summarizes all the RCTs comparing different submucosal injection solutions for colon polypectomy.

Table 7.3 Randomized controlled trials comparing different submucosal injection solutions for colon polypectomy

Study, year	Country	Period	Treatment	Polyp size (mm)	En bloc resection rate	Bleeding rate
Lee, 2007 [19]	Korea	2003–2004	A: Epinephrine-NS (244) B: NS (242)	A: 14.5 ± 5.7 B: 15 ± 6.8	A: 261 (94.9%) B: 268 (93.7%)	A: 12 (4.9%) B: 25 (10.4%)
Katsinelos, 2008 [36]	Greece	2005–2007	A: 50% Dextrose (45) B: Epinephrine-NS (47)	< 20 mm: A: 21 (46.6%) B: 19 (40.4%) 20–39 mm: A: 16 (35.5%) B: 16 (34%) ≥40 mm: A: 8 (17.7%) B: 12 (25.5%)	A: 31 (66.6%) B: 21 (44.7%)	A: 4 (8.8%) B: 5 (10.6%)
Hurlstone, 2008 [37]	UK	NR	A: 50% Dextrose (82) B: Sodium Hyaluronate (81)	A: 18 mm B: 20 mm	A: 59 (72%) B: 56 (69%)	A: 1 (1.2%) B: 4 (4.9%)
Kishihara, 2012 [7]	Japan	2009	A: Sodium Hyaluronate (46) B: NS (48)	A: 11.3 ± 3 B: 12.5 ± 4	A: 45 (98%) B: 45 (94%)	A: 3 (7%) B: 3 (6%)
Yoshida, 2012 [49]	Japan	NR	A: HA (93) B: NS (96)	A: 8.9 (8–16) B: 8.2 (5–15)	A: 90 (96.7%) B: 94 (97.9%)	A: 1 (1.1%) B: 1 (1%)
Moss, 2010 [63]	Australia	2009	A: SG (41) B: NS (39)	A: 40 (25–45) B: 35 (30–50)	A: 12 (30%) B: 6 (15%)	A: 3 (7%) B: 7 (18%)
Fasoulas, 2012 [82]	Greece	2006–2012	A: Epinephrine-HES (25) B: Epinephrine-NS (24)	All LSTs >30 mm	A: 6 (24%) B: 5 (20.8%)	A: 1 (4%) B: 6 (25%)

HA hyaluronic acid, *HES* hydroxyethyl starch, *LST* lateral spreading tumor, *NR* not reported, *NS* normal saline, *SG* succinylated gelatin

All these solutions, despite the promising results in animal/in vitro studies, need to be tested in clinical trials with adequate sample size in order to be introduced in the clinical practice.

Conclusion

Although submucosal injection is not essential for all polypectomy procedures, it is an integral part of injection-assisted EMR. Various solutions have been tested and are currently used, but definitive evidences on the superiority of one submucosal agent over the others are still lacking.

Which particular features of a mucosal lesion determine the real need of submucosal injection and which injection solution is superior are still matter of debate. Addressing this point through adequately sized RCTs represents a pressing need in order to deliver unequivocal guidelines in this important field.

References

1. Winawer SJ, Zauber AG, Ho MN, O'Brien MJ, Gottlieb LS, Sternberg SS, Waye JD, Schapiro M, Bond JH, Panish JF. Prevention of colorectal cancer by colonoscopic polypectomy. The National Polyp Study Workgroup. N Engl J Med. 1993;329:1977–81.
2. Brenner H, Chang-Claude J, Seiler CM, Rickert A, Hoffmeister M. Protection from colorectal cancer after colonoscopy: a population-based, case-control study. Ann Intern Med. 2011;154:22–30.
3. Kedia P, Waye JD. Routine and advanced polypectomy techniques. Curr Gastroenterol Rep. 2011;13:506–11.
4. Kaltenbach T, Soetikno R. Endoscopic resection of large colon polyps. Gastrointest Endosc Clin N Am. 2013;23(1):137–52.
5. Kantsevoy SV, Adler DG, Conway JD, Diehl DL, Farraye FA, Kwon R, Mamula P, Rodriguez S, Shah RJ, Wong Kee Song LM, Tierney WM. Endoscopic mucosal resection and endoscopic submucosal dissection. Gastrointest Endosc. 2008;68:11–8.
6. Jung YK, Park DI. Submucosal injection solutions for endoscopic mucosal resection and endoscopic submucosal dissection of gastrointestinal neoplasms. Gastrointest Interv. 2013;2:73–7.
7. Kishihara T, Chino A, Uragami N, Yoshizawa N, Imai M, Ogawa T, Igarashi M. Usefulness of sodium hyaluronate solution in colorectal endoscopic mucosal resection. Dig Endosc. 2012;24(5):348–52.
8. Al-Taie OH, Bauer Y, Dietrich CG, Fischbach W. Efficacy of submucosal injection of different solutions inclusive blood components on mucosa elevation for endoscopic resection. Clin Exp Gastroenterol. 2012;5:43–8.
9. Holt BA, Bourke MJ. Wide field endoscopic resection for advanced colonic mucosal neoplasia: current status and future directions. Clin Gastroenterol Hepatol. 2012;10(9):969–79.
10. Ngamruengphong S, Pohl H, Haito-Chavez Y, Khashab MA. Update on difficult polypectomy techniques. Curr Gastroenterol Rep. 2016;18(1):3.
11. Uraoka T, Saito Y, Yamamoto K, Fujii T. Submucosal injection solution for gastrointestinal tract endoscopic mucosal resection and endoscopic submucosal dissection. Drug Des Devel Ther. 2009;2:131–8.
12. Yandrapu H, Desai M, Siddique S, Vennalaganti P, Vennalaganti S, Parasa S, Rai T, Kanakadandi V, Bansal A, Titi M, Repici A, Bechtold ML, Sharma P, Choudhary A. Normal saline solution versus other viscous solutions for submucosal injection during endoscopic mucosal resection: a systematic review and meta-analysis. Gastrointest Endosc. 2016;85(4):693–9. in press

13. Tanaka M, Ono H, Hasuike N, Takizawa K. Endoscopic submucosal dissection of early gastric cancer. Digestion. 2008;77(Suppl 1):23–8.
14. Kim SY, Han SH, Kim KH, Kim SO, Han SY, Lee SW, Baek YH. Gastric ischemia after epinephrine injection in a patient with liver cirrhosis. World J Gastroenterol. 2013;19:411–4.
15. Stevens PD, Lebwohl O. Hypertensive emergency and ventricular tachycardia after endoscopic epinephrine injection of a Mallory-Weiss tear. Gastrointest Endosc. 1994;40:77–8.
16. von Delius S, Thies P, Umgelter A, Prinz C, Schmid RM, Huber W. Hemodynamics after endoscopic submucosal injection of epinephrine in patients with nonvariceal upper gastrointestinal bleeding: a matter of concern. Endoscopy. 2006;38:1284–8.
17. Folwaczny C, Heldwein W, Obermaier G, Schindlbeck N. Influence of prophylactic local administration of epinephrine on bleeding complications after polypectomy. Endoscopy. 1997;29(1):31–3.
18. Hsieh YH, Lin HJ, Tseng GY, Perng CL, Li AF, Chang FY, Lee SD. Is submucosal epinephrine injection necessary before polypectomy? A prospective, comparative study. Hepato-Gastroenterology. 2001;48:1379–82.
19. Lee SH, Chung IK, Kim SJ, Kim JO, Ko BM, Kim WH, Kim HS, Park DI, Kim HJ, Byeon JS, Yang SK, Jang BI, Jung SA, Jeen YT, Choi JH, Choi H, Han DS, Song JS. Comparison of postpolypectomy bleeding between epinephrine and saline submucosal injection for large colon polyps by conventional polypectomy: a prospective randomized, multicenter study. World J Gastroenterol. 2007;13(21):2973–7.
20. Corte CJ, Burger DC, Horgan G, Bailey AA, East JE. Postpolypectomy haemorrhage following removal of large polyps using mechanical haemostasis or epinephrine: a meta-analysis. United European Gastroenterol J. 2014;2(2):123–30.
21. Park CH, Jung YS, Nam E, Eun CS, Park DI, Han DS. Comparison of efficacy of prophylactic endoscopic therapies for postpolypectomy bleeding in the colorectum: a systematic review and network meta-analysis. Am J Gastroenterol. 2016;111(9):1230–43.
22. Rohde H, Guenther MW, Budde R, Mühlhofer H. Randomized trial of prophylactic epinephrine-saline injection before snare polypectomy to prevent bleeding. Endoscopy. 2000;32:1004–5.
23. Di Giorgio P, De Luca L, Calcagno G, Rivellini G, Mandato M, De Luca B. Detachable snare versus epinephrine injection in the prevention of postpolypectomy bleeding: a randomized and controlled study. Endoscopy. 2004;36:860–3.
24. Dobrowolski S, Dobosz M, Babicki A, Dymecki D, Hać S. Prophylactic submucosal saline adrenaline injection in colonoscopic polypectomy: prospective randomized study. Surg Endosc. 2004;18:990–3.
25. Paspatis GA, Paraskeva K, Theodoropoulou A, Mathou N, Vardas E, Oustamanolakis P, Chlouverakis G, Karagiannis I. A prospective, randomized comparison of adrenaline injection in combination with detachable snare versus adrenaline injection alone in the prevention of postpolypectomy bleeding in large colonic polyps. Am J Gastroenterol. 2006;101:2805.
26. Kouklakis G, Mpoumponaris A, Gatopoulou A, Efraimidou E, Manolas K, Lirantzopoulos N. Endoscopic resection of large pedunculated colonic polyps and risk of postpolypectomy bleeding with adrenaline injection versus endoloop and hemoclip: a prospective, randomized study. Surg Endosc. 2009;23:2732–7.
27. Holt BA, Jayasekeran V, Sonson R, Bourke MJ. Topical submucosal chromoendoscopy defines the level of resection in colonic EMR and may improve procedural safety (with video). Gastrointest Endosc. 2013;77:949–53.
28. Fujishiro M, Yahagi N, Kashimura K, Mizushima Y, Oka M, Enomoto S, Kakushima N, Kobayashi K, Hashimoto T, Iguchi M, Shimizu Y, Ichinose M, Omata M. Comparison of various submucosal injection solutions for maintaining mucosal elevation during endoscopic mucosal resection. Endoscopy. 2004;36:579–83.
29. Fujishiro M, Yahagi N, Kashimura K, Matsuura T, Nakamura M, Kakushima N, Kodashima S, Ono S, Kobayashi K, Hashimoto T, Yamamichi N, Tateishi A, Shimizu Y, Oka M, Ichinose M, Omata M. Tissue damage of different submucosal injection solutions for EMR. Gastrointest Endosc. 2005;62:933–42.

30. Sakamaki M, Igarashi H, Nishiyama Y, Hagiwara H, Ando J, Chishiki T, Curran BC, Katayama Y. Effect of glycerol on ischemic cerebral edema assessed by magnetic resonance imaging. J Neurol Sci. 2003;209:69–74.
31. Torii A, Sakai M, Kajiyama T, Kishimoto H, Kin G, Inoue K, Koizumi T, Ueda S, Okuma M. Endoscopic aspiration mucosectomy as curative endoscopic surgery: analysis of 24 cases of early gastric cancer. Gastrointest Endosc. 1995;42:475–9.
32. Sumiyoshi T, Fujii T, Sumiyoshi Y. Injected substances to the submucosa in endoscopic mucosal resection: glycerin solution versus normal saline solution. Gastrointest Endosc. 2002;55:AB110.
33. Uraoka T, Fujii T, Saito Y, Sumiyoshi T, Emura F, Bhandari P, Matsuda T, Fu KI, Saito D. Effectiveness of glycerol as a submucosal injection for EMR. Gastrointest Endosc. 2005;61:736–40.
34. Varadarajulu S, Tamhane A, Slaughter RL. Evaluation of dextrose 50% as a medium for injection-assisted polypectomy. Endoscopy. 2006;38:907–12.
35. Katsinelos P, Kountouras J, Paroutoglou G, Chatzimavroudis G, Zavos C, Pilpilidis I, Gelas G, Paikos D, Karakousis K. A comparative study of 50% dextrose and normal saline solution on their ability to create submucosal fluid cushions for endoscopic resection of sessile rectosigmoid polyps. Gastrointest Endosc. 2008;68:692–8.
36. Katsinelos P, Kountouras J, Paroutoglou G, Zavos C, Rizos C, Beltsis A. Endoscopic mucosal resection of large sessile colorectal polyps with submucosal injection of hypertonic 50 percent dextrose-epinephrine solution. Dis Colon Rectum. 2006;49:1384–92.
37. Hurlstone DP, Fu KI, Brown SR, Thomson M, Atkinson R, Tiffin N, Cross SS. EMR using dextrose solution versus sodium hyaluronate for colorectal Paris type I and 0-II lesions: a randomized endoscopist-blinded study. Endoscopy. 2008;40(2):110–4.
38. Ferreira AO, Moleiro J, Torres J, Dinis-Ribeiro M. Solutions for submucosal injection in endoscopic resection: a systematic review and meta-analysis. Endosc Int Open. 2016;4(1):E1–E16.
39. Hwang JH, Konda V, Abu Dayyeh BK, Chauhan SS, Enestvedt BK, Fujii-Lau LL, Komanduri S, Maple JT, Murad FM, Pannala R, Thosani NC, Banerjee S. Endoscopic mucosal resection. Gastrointest Endosc. 2015;82(2):215–26.
40. Santilli V, Paoloni M, Mangone M, Alviti F, Bernetti A. Hyaluronic acid in the management of osteoarthritis: injection therapies innovations. Clin Cases Miner Bone Metab. 2016;13(2):131–4.
41. Robert L. Hyaluronan, a truly "youthful" polysaccharide. Its medical applications. Pathol Biol (Paris). 2015;63(1):32–4.
42. Yoshida N, Naito Y, Kugai M, Inoue K, Uchiyama K, Takagi T, Ishikawa T, Handa O, Konishi H, Wakabayashi N, Yagi N, Kokura S, Morimoto Y, Kanemasa K, Yanagisawa A, Yoshikawa T. Efficacy of hyaluronic acid in endoscopic mucosal resection of colorectal tumors. J Gastroenterol Hepatol. 2011;26:286–91.
43. Hyun JJ, Chun HR, Jeen YT, Baeck CW, Yu SK, Kim YS, Lee HS, Um SH, Lee SW, Choi JH, Kim CD, Ryu HS, Hyun JH. Comparison of the characteristics of submucosal injection solutions used in endoscopic mucosal resection. Scand J Gastroenterol. 2006;41:488–92.
44. Yamamoto H, Yube T, Isoda N, Sato Y, Sekine Y, Higashizawa T, Ido K, Kimura K, Kanai N. A novel method of endoscopic mucosal resection using sodium hyaluronate. Gastrointest Endosc. 1999;50:251–6.
45. Yamamoto H, Kawata H, Sunada K, Satoh K, Kaneko Y, Ido K, Sugano K. Success rate of curative endoscopic mucosal resection with circumferential mucosal incision assisted by submucosal injection of sodium hyaluronate. Gastrointest Endosc. 2002;56:507–12.
46. Yamamoto H, Kawata H, Sunada K, Sasaki A, Nakazawa K, Miyata T, Sekine Y, Yano T, Satoh K, Ido K, Sugano K. Successful en-bloc resection of large superficial tumors in the stomach and colon using sodium hyaluronate and small-caliber-tip transparent hood. Endoscopy. 2003;35:690–4.
47. Hirasaki S, Kozu T, Yamamoto H, Sano Y, Yahagi N, Oyama T, Shimoda T, Sugano K, Tajiri H, Takekoshi T, Saito D. Usefulness and safety of 0.4% sodium hyaluronate solution as a submucosal fluid "cushion" for endoscopic resection of colorectal mucosal neoplasms: a prospective multicenter open-label trial. BMC Gastroenterol. 2009;9:1.
48. Yamamoto H, Yahagi N, Oyama T, Gotoda T, Doi T, Hirasaki S, Shimoda T, Sugano K, Tajiri H, Takekoshi T, Saito D. Usefulness and safety of 0.4% sodium hyaluronate solution as a

submucosal fluid "cushion" in endoscopic resection for gastric neoplasms: a prospective multicenter trial. Gastrointest Endosc. 2008;67:830–9.

49. Yoshida N, Naito Y, Inada Y, Kugai M, Kamada K, Katada K, Uchiyama K, Ishikawa T, Takagi T, Handa O, Konishi H, Yagi N, Kokura S, Wakabayashi N, Yanagisawa A, Yoshikawa T. Endoscopic mucosal resection with 0.13% hyaluronic acid solution for colorectal polyps less than 20 mm: a randomized controlled trial. J Gastroenterol Hepatol. 2012;27(8):1377–83.

50. Saito Y, Emura F, Matsuda T, Uraoka T, Nakajima T, Ikematsu H, Gotoda T, Saito D, Fujii T. A new sinker-assisted endoscopic submucosal dissection for colorectal cancer. Gastrointest Endosc. 2005;62:297–301.

51. Kim ER, Park YG, Min BH, Lee JH, Rhee PL, Kim JJ, Park JH, Park DI, Chang DK. Usefulness of ready-to-use 0.4% sodium hyaluronate (endo-ease) in the endoscopic resection of gastrointestinal neoplasms. Clin Endosc. 2015;48(5):392–8.

52. Matsui Y, Inomata M, Izumi K, Sonoda K, Shiraishi N, Kitano S. Hyaluronic acid stimulates tumor-cell proliferation at wound sites. Gastrointest Endosc. 2004;60:539–43.

53. Fujishiro M, Yahagi N, Kashimura K, Mizushima Y, Oka M, Matsuura T, Enomoto S, Kakushima N, Imagawa A, Kobayashi K, Hashimoto T, Iguchi M, Shimizu Y, Ichinose M, Omata M. Different mixtures of sodium hyaluronate and their ability to create submucosal fluid cushions for endoscopic mucosal resection. Endoscopy. 2004;36:584–9.

54. Fujishiro M, Yahagi N, Nakamura M, Kakushima N, Kodashima S, Ono S, Kobayashi K, Hashimoto T, Yamamichi N, Tateishi A, Shimizu Y, Oka M, Ogura K, Kawabe T, Ichinose M, Omata M. Successful outcomes of a novel endoscopic treatment for GI tumors: endoscopic submucosal dissection with a mixture of high-molecular-weight hyaluronic acid, glycerin, and sugar. Gastrointest Endosc. 2006;63:243–9.

55. Friedland S, Kothari S, Chen A, Park W, Banerjee S. Endoscopic mucosal resection with an over-the-counter hyaluronate preparation. Gastrointest Endosc. 2012;75(5):1040–4.

56. Lee SH, Cho WY, Kim HJ, Kim HJ, Kim YH, Chung IK, Kim HS, Park SH, Kim SJ. A new method of EMR: submucosal injection of a fibrinogen mixture. Gastrointest Endosc. 2004;59:220–4.

57. Lee SH, Park JH, Park do H, Chung IK, Kim HS, Park SH, Kim SJ, Cho HD. Clinical efficacy of EMR with submucosal injection of a fibrinogen mixture: a prospective randomized trial. Gastrointest Endosc. 2006;64:691–6.

58. Ravalico G, Tognetto D, Baccara F, Lovisato A. Corneal endothelial protection by different viscoelastics during phacoemulsification. J Cataract Refract Surg. 1997;23:433–9.

59. Feitoza AB, Gostout CJ, Burgart LJ, Burkert A, Herman LJ, Rajan E. Hydroxypropyl methylcellulose: a better submucosal fluid cushion for endoscopic mucosal resection. Gastrointest Endosc. 2003;57:41–7.

60. Rajan E, Gostout CJ, Feitoza AB, Leontovich ON, Herman LJ, Burgart LJ, Chung S, Cotton PB, Hawes RH, Kalloo AN, Kantsevoy SV, Pasricha PJ. Widespread EMR: a new technique for removal of large areas of mucosa. Gastrointest Endosc. 2004;60:623–7.

61. Lenz L, Di Sena V, Nakao FS, de Andrade GP, Rohr MR, Ferrari AP Jr. Comparative results of gastric submucosal injection with hydroxypropyl methylcellulose, carboxymethylcellulose and normal saline solution in a porcine model. Arq Gastroenterol. 2010;47:184–7.

62. Moss A, Bourke MJ, Kwan V, Tran K, Godfrey C, McKay G, Hopper AD. Succinylated gelatin substantially increases en bloc resection size in colonic EMR: a randomized, blinded trial in a porcine model. Gastrointest Endosc. 2010;71(3):589–95.

63. Moss A, Bourke MJ, Metz AJ. A randomized, double-blind trial of succinylated gelatin submucosal injection for endoscopic resection of large sessile polyps of the colon. Am J Gastroenterol. 2010;105(11):2375–82.

64. Robertson CS, Womack C, Robson K, Morris DL. A study of the local toxicity of agents used for variceal injection sclerotherapy. HPB Surg. 1989;1:149–54.

65. Facciorusso A, Di Maso M, Antonino M, Del Prete V, Panella C, Barone M, Muscatiello N. Polidocanol injection decreases the bleeding rate after colon polypectomy: a propensity score analysis. Gastrointest Endosc. 2015;82(2):350–8.

66. Repici A, Pohl H. Revival of a sclerosing agent for prevention of postpolypectomy bleeding. Gastrointest Endosc. 2015;82(2):359–61.

67. Muscatiello N, Facciorusso A. Use of polidocanol in colon polypectomy. Gastrointest Endosc. 2016;83(1):271.
68. Giday SA, Magno P, Buscaglia JM, Canto MI, Ko CW, Shin EJ, Xia L, Wroblewski LM, Clarke JO, Kalloo AN, Jagannath SB, Kantsevoy SV. Is blood the ideal submucosal cushioning agent? A comparative study in a porcine model. Endoscopy. 2006;38:1230–4.
69. Shastri YM, Kriener S, Caspary WF, Schneider A. Autologous blood as a submucosal fluid cushion for endoscopic mucosal therapies: results of an ex vivo study. Scand J Gastroenterol. 2007;42:1369–75.
70. Sato T. A novel method of endoscopic mucosal resection assisted by submucosal injection of autologous blood (blood patch EMR). Dis Colon Rectum. 2006;49:1636–41.
71. Fredericks CM, Kotry I, Holtz G, Askalani AH, Serour GI. Adhesion prevention in the rabbit with sodium carboxymethylcellulose solutions. Am J Obstet Gynecol. 1986;155(3):667–70.
72. Burns JW, Colt MJ, Burgees LS, Skinner KC. Preclinical evaluation of Seprafilm bioresorbable membrane. Eur J Surg Suppl. 1997;577:40–8.
73. Yamasaki M, Kume K, Yoshikawa I, Otsuki M. A novel method of endoscopic submucosal dissection with blunt abrasion by submucosal injection of sodium carboxymethylcellulose: an animal preliminary study. Gastrointest Endosc. 2006;64(6):958–65.
74. Ishihara M, Ono K, Sato M, Nakanishi K, Saito Y, Yura H, Matsui T, Hattori H, Fujita M, Kikuchi M, Kurita A. Acceleration of wound contraction and healing with a photocrosslinkable chitosan hydrogel. Wound Repair Regen. 2001;9(6):513–21.
75. Ono K, Saito Y, Yura H, Ishikawa K, Kurita A, Akaike T, Ishihara M. Photocrosslinkable chitosan as a biological adhesive. J Biomed Mater Res. 2000;49(2):289–95.
76. Ishizuka T, Hayashi T, Ishihara M, Yoshizumi Y, Aiko S, Nakamura S, Yura H, Kanatani Y, Nogami Y, Maehara T. Submucosal injection, for endoscopic mucosal resection, of photocrosslinkable chitosan hydrogel in DMEM/F12 medium. Endoscopy. 2007;39(5):428–33.
77. Ishizuka T, Ishihara M, Aiko S, Nogami Y, Nakamura S, Kanatani Y, Kishimoto S, Hattori H, Horio T, Tanaka Y, Maehara T. Experimental evaluation of photocrosslinkable chitosan hydrogel as injection solution for endoscopic resection. Endoscopy. 2009;41(1):25–8.
78. Tran RT, Palmer M, Tang SJ, Abell TL, Yang J. Injectable drug-eluting elastomeric polymer: a novel submucosal injection material. Gastrointest Endosc. 2012;75(5):1092–7.
79. Eun SH, Cho JY, Jung IS, Ko BM, Hong SJ, Ryu CB, Kim JO, Jin SY, Lee JS, Lee MS, Shim CS, Kim BS. Effectiveness of sodium alginate as a submucosal injection material for endoscopic mucosal resection in animal. Gut Liver. 2007;1(1):27–32.
80. Kang KJ, Min BH, Lee JH, Kim ER, Sung CO, Cho JY, Seo SW, Kim JJ. Alginate hydrogel as a potential alternative to hyaluronic acid as submucosal injection material. Dig Dis Sci. 2013;58(6):1491–6.
81. Akagi T, Yasuda K, Tajima M, Suzuki K, Inomata M, Shiraishi N, Sato Y, Kitano S. Sodium alginate as an ideal submucosal injection material for endoscopic submucosal resection: preliminary experimental and clinical study. Gastrointest Endosc. 2011;74(5):1026–32.
82. Fasoulas K, Lazaraki G, Chatzimavroudis G, Paroutoglou G, Katsinelos T, Dimou E, Geros C, Zavos C, Kountouras J, Katsinelos P. Endoscopic mucosal resection of giant laterally spreading tumors with submucosal injection of hydroxyethyl starch: comparative study with normal saline solution. Surg Laparosc Endosc Percutan Tech. 2012;22(3):272–8.

Management of Complications After Endoscopic Polypectomy

8

Valentina Del Prete, Matteo Antonino,
Rosario Vincenzo Buccino, Nicola Muscatiello,
and Antonio Facciorusso

8.1   Introduction

Polypectomy is associated with complications such as bleeding, perforation, and post-polypectomy coagulation syndrome that is extremely rare. Additionally, one third of patients report gastrointestinal symptoms including abdominal pain, diarrhea, bloating, and nausea that resolve within 24–48 h.

As for post-polypectomy bleeding and perforation, data from the English National Health Service Bowel Cancer Screening Programme (NHSBCSP) report an 11-fold and threefold increased risk as compared to diagnostic colonoscopy [1]; hence the proper management of these common complications should be part of the background knowledge of every endoscopist.

8.2   Post-polypectomy Bleeding (PPB)

Post-polypectomy bleeding (PPB) may occur immediately or may be delayed (from days to week after the procedure).

Immediate or intra-procedural bleeding occurs during the procedure and persists for more than 60 s or requires endoscopic treatment. Delayed or post-procedural bleeding occurs after the procedure, up to 30 days post-polypectomy [2].

Many studies have identified a risk of PPB ranging from 0.07 to 1.7% [3–5]. Data from the English National Health Service Bowel Cancer Screening Programme on 69.028 polypectomies found an overall PPB rate of 1.14% [1]. Intra-procedural bleeding occurs in 2.8% of standard polypectomies [6], while delayed

V. Del Prete (✉) • M. Antonino • R. Vincenzo Buccino • N. Muscatiello • A. Facciorusso
Gastroenterology Unit, Department of Medical Sciences, University of Foggia,
AOU Ospedali Riuniti, Viale Pinto, 1, 71100 Foggia, Italy
e-mail: valedelprete80@gmail.com

© Springer International Publishing AG 2018
A. Facciorusso, N. Muscatiello (eds.), *Colon Polypectomy*,
https://doi.org/10.1007/978-3-319-59457-6_8

(post-procedural) bleeding varies from 0.6 to 2.2% in large series (>1000 polypectomies) [7–9].

Endoscopic mucosal resection (EMR) of small lesions (<10 mm) is associated with PPB rates similar to those of conventional polypectomy. In large series of EMR (>1000 cases) which reported higher rates of PPB, the incidence ranges between 3.7 and 11.3% for immediate PPB and 0.6–6.2% for delayed PPB [10–12].

Endoscopic submucosal dissection (ESD) was found to present an overall bleeding rate of 2% in a recent meta-analysis [13]. Another recent meta-analysis of eight studies including 2299 colorectal lesions showed lower rate of delayed PPB for ESD compared with EMR (OR 0.85, 95% CI 0.45–1.60) [14].

8.2.1 Risk Factors for PPB

8.2.1.1 Polyp-Related Factors
Polyp-related factors are size, location, and morphology. Polyp size is the most important risk factor for PPB and every −1 mm increase in diameter leads to an augmented risk of bleeding of 9% for polyps greater than 1 cm [15]. Overall, polyps larger than 1 cm have a twofold to 4.5-fold increased risk of bleeding [16, 17].

Other additional baseline predictive factors for bleeding are location in the right hemicolon (2.6-fold to 4.6-fold risk) [18, 19], pedunculated polyps (with a stalk diameter >5 mm) [20], and laterally spreading tumors (LST) [16, 17]. In an Australian prospective multicenter study of 1172 patients with LST with mean size 35.5 mm, intra-procedural bleeding was experienced in 11.3% of cases and was associated with increasing size, villous or tubular-villous histology, Paris type 0–IIa + Is lesions, and low-volume centers with less than 75 EMR performed. In the same study, delayed PPB occurred in 6.2% of cases and was associated with proximal colon location (OR 3.72), use of electrosurgical current not controlled by a microprocessor (OR 2.03), and immediate PPB (OR 2.16) [10].

In some studies polyp pathology resulted as a risk factor for PPB with villous features or adenocarcinoma at higher bleeding risk [9, 16, 21]. In a recent prospective study on 15,553 polypectomies from 2005 to 2013, hamartomatous polyps (juvenile and Peutz-Jeghers polyps) resulted as a risk factor for delayed hemorrhage with odds ratios of 5.7 and 4.3 as compared to inflammatory/hyperplastic polyps [22].

8.2.1.2 Patient-Related Factors
Age greater than 65 years, hypertension, cardiac disease, renal disease, and antithrombotic therapy have been associated with a higher risk for PPB [17, 21]. In a recent study, patients with BMI > 25 kg/m^2 had 3.7 times higher risk of delayed PPB than those with BMI <25 kg/m^2 [23].

The use of antithrombotic therapy is one of the major risk factors for PPB; risk varies based on the type of antithrombotic agent (antiplatelet agent or anticoagulant) [24].

Antiplatelet agents (APA) are aspirin and thienopyridines (clopidogrel, ticagrelor, prasugrel).

Despite the well-known bleeding risk related to aspirin use [25–27], however most data shows that aspirin use is safe and does not increase the risk of PPB [28, 29]. Therefore, both the European and the American guidelines recommend continuing aspirin in patients undergoing polypectomy, while the BSG-ESGE guidelines recommend discontinuing aspirin in the case of EDS and large colonic EMR (>20 mm) [24].

A recent meta-analysis of five observational studies found that continued therapy with clopidogrel increases the risk of delayed but not immediate post-polypectomy bleeding [30] with an overall pooled relative risk (RR) for PPB of 2.54 ($p < 0.5$). Other studies confirm the increased risk of delayed PPB in patients in therapy with clopidogrel [25]. No data are available on PPB in patients taking other thienopyridines.

American and European guidelines recommend discontinuation of thienopyridines 5 days before polypectomy when the thrombotic risk is low, while in patients on dual antiplatelet therapy (DAPT), continuation of aspirin is suggested. In the case of high thrombotic risk, current guidelines recommend continuing aspirin and liaising with a cardiologist about the discontinuation of thienopyridines [24, 31].

Patients anticoagulated with warfarin have a significantly increased risk of PPB; hence it is recommended that patients at low thrombotic risk should discontinue warfarin 5 days before polypectomy reaching a value of INR < 1.5 and restart therapy on the day of the procedure [24, 31]. Patients at high thrombotic risk should substitute warfarin with low molecular weight heparin (LMWH).

No data on PPB in patients taking DOAC (direct oral anticoagulant) are currently available. In these patients is recommended discontinuation of therapy 48 h before the procedure [24, 31].

8.2.1.3 Technique-Related Factors

Polyps less than 10 mm can be removed with biopsy forceps, cold snare, and hot snare.

Cold forceps biopsy polypectomy is the simplest method, but it is associated with significant rates of incomplete polyp removal.

Snare polypectomy can be cold or hot if supplemented by electrocautery. A prospective multicenter trial of 1015 polyps (<10 mm) removed with cold techniques (biopsy forceps or snare) found that these techniques are safe and associated with an increased risk of intra-procedural bleeding but not of delayed PPB; bleeding was successfully treated by endoscopic hemostasis in all cases without further medical intervention [8].

Cold snare polypectomy is considered the technique of choice for polyps less than 10 mm; in two studies [32, 33] intra-procedural bleeding was more frequent in the case of cold snare polypectomy but resolved without intervention, while in another study intra-procedural and delayed PPB was more frequently reported in hot snare polypectomy group [33, 34]. All these studies concluded that cold snare polypectomy is superior to hot snare, quicker, and with less post-procedural abdominal symptoms.

Electrocautery is used to remove polyps greater than 10 mm; electrosurgical settings used for snare resection are pure coagulation, cutting, and blended current [35].

Table 8.1 Risk factors for post-polypectomy bleeding (PPB)

Polyp-related factors	Patient-related factors	Technique-related factors
- Size (>1 cm) - Location (right colon) - Morphology (pedunculated polyps, LST) - Pathology (villous, tubular-villous, hamartomatous polyps)	- Age <65 - Hypertension - Cardiac disease - Renal disease - Antithrombotic therapy - BMI < 25 kg/m^2	- Hot snare polypectomy - Electrocautery

The use of cutting and blended current has been associated with immediate PPB, whereas the use of coagulation current has been associated with delayed PPB [36].

Main risk factors for post-polypectomy bleeding are reported in Table 8.1.

8.2.2 Management of PPB

The available options to treat PPB are injectable solutions and thermal and mechanical devices.

For intra-procedural bleeding, endoscopic coagulation (snare-tip soft coagulation or coagulation forceps) or mechanical therapy (endoclips) is recommended, with or without injection of diluted adrenaline solution (1:10,000 or 1:20,000) [2]. Application of through-the-scope clips is one of the most used methods; in the case of bleeding after the removal of a sessile polyp, clip must be placed directly over the point of bleeding opposing the mucosa on both sides, while if the bleeding is from the stump of a pedunculated polyp, clips should be placed perpendicular to the stalk base. The snare-tip soft coagulation is a technique that involves protruding the snare tip beyond the catheter, followed by application of coagulating current while touching the tip directly onto the bleeding point. Coagulation forceps are reserved for more complicated and severe cases [37]. Adrenaline injection can be useful to obtain initial control of hemorrhage, but it should be always used in combination with other techniques. Washing with a foot pedal-controlled water pump is useful to clear the field, to point the bleeding vessel, and to confirm the cessation of bleeding after the treatment. Washing also infiltrates the submucosal tissue inducing a tamponade effect [38].

Over-the-scope clips (OTSC; Ovesco Endoscopy, Tuebingen, Germany) are effective in the case of refractory bleeding [39, 40].

In the case of delayed PPB if patient is hemodynamically stable and with no ongoing hemorrhage, a conservative management is recommended [2]; in >50% of cases, bleeding stops spontaneously and does not require any intervention. If bleeding persists patient should repeat colonoscopy, after an adequate bowel preparation in order to identify the site of active bleeding. Endoscopic treatment with forceps coagulation or mechanical therapy with or without adrenaline injection is recommended [41]. There is no consensus on the technique of choice, but the most commonly used methods are clipping and forceps coagulation (with or without adrenaline injections). Clipping has been found to be superior to forceps coagulation especially because it limits tissue injury [42]. Some studies have shown efficacy of band ligation to treat PPB in the case of pedunculated or semi-pedunculated polyps [43].

Intra-procedural bleeding after EMR is usually controlled by thermal devices and the use of a voltage-limited microprocessor to prevent deep thermal injury. In particular, snare-tip soft coagulation is an effective method to control bleeding during EMR [41]. If this technique does not achieve hemostasis, additional treatments with endoclips or coagulation forceps are recommended [44]. Delayed PPB is managed as previously described.

In the case of ESD, risk factors for bleeding are lesion size (>30 mm), rectal location of lesions, presence of submucosal fibrosis, and low-volume centers [45, 46]. Intra-procedural bleeding can be managed using settings on the electrosurgical unit during the precut and submucosal dissection phases. Bleeding during dissection can be treated by soft coagulation followed by application of the coagulation grasper to the bleeding vessel if hemostasis with the former method is unsuccessful. Delayed bleeding can be treated with conventional endoscopic techniques, preferably with endoclips to avoid worsening of thermal injury [47].

8.2.3 Prevention of PPB

There is no consensus on the prophylaxis of PPB.

Epinephrine injection is associated with lower rates of PPB compared with saline injection or no injection [48, 49]. We evaluated the efficacy of submucosal injection of polidocanol in the prophylaxis of PPB compared to epinephrine solution injection in a series of 612 patients with large sessile polyps (>20 mm). Polidocanol resulted more effective than epinephrine in preventing both immediate and delayed post-polypectomy bleeding (3.9% vs 10.7% of control group, $p = 0.001$ and 1.3% vs 6.2% of control group, $p = 0.002$, respectively) [50].

Prophylactic clip placement is ineffective in reducing delayed bleeding in polyps <10 mm in size [51]. On the other hand, in a retrospective study of 524 polyps >20 mm, prophylactic clipping was associated with a reduced risk of PPB [52].

Prophylactic clipping after standard polypectomy or EMR may be considered on the basis of patient and polyp-related risk factors and reserved to patients at high risk of post-polypectomy bleeding [2], but more RCTs on prophylactic therapies are required.

A meta-analysis and systematic review found that both monotherapy (epinephrine injection or clip placement) and combined therapy (epinephrine injection and clip placement) reduce immediate PPB, whereas combination therapy is superior to monotherapy in the prevention of immediate PPB. Monotherapy with mechanical devices and combined therapy are effective in the prevention of delayed PPB, while monotherapy with epinephrine injection is ineffective [53].

Cautery is useful to treat PPB, but neither argon plasma coagulation (APC) nor coagulation forceps have been effective in the prevention of post-polypectomy bleeding [54, 55].

8.3   Colon Perforation

Colon perforation (CP) is widely recognized as one of the most serious post-polypectomy complications. The rates range from 0.01 to 0.8% for diagnostic colonoscopy but can reach 5% following therapeutic procedures, such as endoscopic submucosal dissection (ESD) [56]. The main consequence of these procedures is the resection of mucosa, thus weakening the colon wall and increasing the risk of perforation and post-polypectomy syndrome [57].

Since colon perforation is a dreaded complication potentially leading to tension pneumoperitoneum (presence of air in to peritoneum) which is responsible for cardiovascular arrest, prophylactic clip closure has been found to be effective in closing the wall breach [58].

Carbon dioxide insufflation and periodic decompression of the colon as well as removing the biopsy cap could also prevent pneumoperitoneum [59, 60].

Once pneumoperitoneum is diagnosed, the treatment consists in drainage by insertion of angiocath or alternatively in leaving the endoscope in the colon to decompress it.

Besides air escape, fecal and fluid leakage out of the colonic wall may occur; hence adequate cleansing is important to avoid peritonitis [60].

Micro-perforation and macro-perforation are distinguished on the base of the size of perforation and the timing of detection (the former is not detected during endoscopy, whereas the latter is easily diagnosed immediately by the endoscopist). They are both result of cautery and dissection of the submucosal layer. Timing of detection is crucial since in the case of immediate diagnosis, endoscopic treatment may be still feasible, while surgery is mandatory when detection of perforation is late.

Risk factors for macro-perforation are the failure of lifting the lesion by injection of submucosal solution, resection into deep submucosa, and attempted polypectomy [59].

8.3.1   Risk Factors for Perforation

Risk factors are mainly related to polyp features and technique/device adopted. Polyp-related factors are location, morphology, and size of lesion. A non-pedunculated polyp in the distal colon is associated with a 12-fold decreased risk of perforation as compared to a similar polyp in the cecum [61]. Likewise, laterally spreading or non-polypoid lesions are at higher risk of perforation. Additionally, the grade of infiltration of lesion in the wall is an independent risk factor (Vienna classification 4, noninvasive high-grade dysplasia, and Vienna classification 5, invasive neoplasia) [62].

Finally, previous polypectomy attempts cause submucosal fibrosis which will impair successful lifting of the lesion with submucosal injection and increase the risk of perforation [63].

The main mechanisms of perforation are mechanical injury (55%), polypectomy (27%), or thermal injury (18%) [64, 65].

Blunt trauma can occur in the attempt to explore a tract of the colon (commonly the sigma) that may be fixed by adhesions or extremely redundant [65].

In addition, retroflexion of the colonoscope, severe proctitis, and pelvic radiation therapy are other recognized risk factors.

Different resection techniques lead to different risks of perforation: 0.01% with hot biopsy, 0.17% with polypectomy, 0.91% with EMR, and 3.3% with ESD [66].

Unlike perforations resulting from mechanical injury and polypectomy, perforations from thermal injuries (due to electrocautery or APC used to ablate tissue or control bleeding) tend to be small (1 cm) and are often located in the cecum [67].

Finally the expertise of the endoscopist influences perforation risk, while deep sedation (with propofol) does not seem to influence it [67, 68].

8.3.2   Prevention of Colon Perforation

Several precautions should be considered before the procedure to reduce the risk of perforation or at least to manage its consequences. First, the patient should always be counseled on benefits and risk especially in the case of complicated polypectomy of larger lesions [69].

Proper bowel preparation is of paramount importance to avoid the ultimate consequence of perforation, namely, fecal peritonitis. In this regard, a split dose of PEG seems to be the protocol of choice [70].

As for polyp resection, the use of distal attachment devices (such as cap-fitted colonoscope) may allow to have an easier approach to lesions hidden between the folds and help to optimize endoclip placement [71].

As previously described, insufflation with carbon dioxide rather than room air may minimize the risk of pneumoperitoneum especially with prolonged procedures, thus reducing post-procedure abdominal pain and hospitalization [72].

8.3.3   Management of Colon Perforation

Proper assessment of the depth of resection and immediate identification of perforation during endoscopy dramatically decrease the need of surgery. Dye solution injection to form cushion underneath the polyp may be useful in these cases since a persistent absence of staining is related to a deep injury and exposed or submucosal fibrosis [73, 74].

The white cautery ring indicating disruption of the muscularis layer resembles a target sign surrounded by blue-stained submucosa. A corresponding target sign will also be present on the underside of the resected specimen [75]. These advances allow early detection of perforation during the procedure before the overt clinical signs or free air seen on radiographic imaging and further stress the importance of methodically examining the polypectomy defect. Full-thickness resections and deep resection with exposure of the muscle should be closed with clips.

Currently available through-the-scope clips (TTSC) allow to rotate and regulate the angle for placement and eventually to reopen if closure is not successful [76]. On the other hand, TTSC present a smaller wingspan and lower closure force, and often multiple clips are needed.

Over-the-scope clips (OTSC) are made of nitinol (nickel–titanium alloy) that fit over the distal tip of endoscope. They can have rounded teeth for hemostasis and pointed teeth to close perforations.

OTSC grasp more tissue than TTSC, but its disadvantage is that it must be loaded on the scope before closing the tip [77–79].

Therefore, TTSC may be of use in the case of wall defect smaller than 2 cm, whereas OTSC should be considered for larger breaches or ESD-related perforations [80].

8.3.4   Patient Management After Perforation

The patient must be promptly hospitalized, and broad-spectrum intravenous antibiotic and fluids should be administered, with blood count monitored every 6–8 h.

To prevent cardiopulmonary compromise, tension pneumoperitoneum should be decompressed using an 18–20 gauge needle [81].

Surgical counseling is strongly suggested even when endoscope closure has been achieved, whereas surgery is mandatory in the case of large perforations or generalized peritonitis. In one series, technical success rate of TTSC closure was 91% (29/32) with seven patients requiring surgery. TTSC was clinically unsuccessful in five patients who finally required surgical intervention [82]. Risk factors associated with the need for early surgical treatment (within 24 h of endoscopic closure) were perforations greater than 1 cm, persistent leukocytosis, fever, severe abdominal pain, and a large amount of free intraperitoneal air (extending more than 3 cm below the diaphragm) [82].

Strict observation is needed after closing the wall defect in order to detect those subjects who develop late complications needing surgery.

With the correct timing and technique, endoscopic treatment of perforation leads to similar results as compared to surgery [83].

8.4   Post-polypectomy Syndrome

Post-polypectomy syndrome is the result of the transmural thermal injury which leads to a peritonitis in the absence of perforation [84], and its incidence varies from 1 in 1000 to 3 per 100,000 examinations.

Non-polypoid morphology, size larger than 1 cm, and hypertension are well-recognized risk factors of post-polypectomy syndrome [85]. Common symptoms are fever, leukocytosis, and localized abdominal pain and tenderness 1–5 days after polypectomy.

The treatment includes fasting, antibiotic for 7 days, and hospitalization for 5 days [84].

References

1. Rutter MD, Nickerson C, Rees CJ, et al. Risk factors for adverse events related to polypectomy in the English bowel cancer screening programme. Endoscopy. 2014;46:90–7.
2. Ferlitsch M, Moss A, Hassan C, Bhandari P, Dumonceau JM, Paspatis G, Jover R, Langner C, Bronzwaer M, Nalankilli K, Fockens P, Hazzan R, Gralnek IM, Gschwantler M, Waldmann E, Jeschek P, Penz D, Heresbach D, Moons L, Lemmers A, Paraskeva K, Pohl J, Ponchon T, Regula J, Repici A, Rutter MD, Burgess NG, Bourke MJ. Colorectal polypectomy and endoscopic mucosal resection (EMR): European Society of Gastrointestinal Endoscopy Clinical Guideline. Endoscopy. 2017;49(3):270–97.
3. Wexner SD, Garbus JE, Singh JJ, SAGES Colonoscopy Study Outcomes group. A prospective analysis of 13.580 colonoscopies. Re-evaluation of credentialing guidelines. Surg Endosc. 2001;15:251–61.
4. Bowles CJ, Leicester R, Romaya C, Swarbrick E, Williams CB, Epstein O. A prospective study of colonoscopy practice in the UK today: are we adequately prepared for national colorectal cancer screening tomorrow? Gut. 2004;53:277–83.
5. Gibbs DH, Opelka FG, Beck DE, Hicks TC, Timmcke AE, Gathright JB Jr. Post-polypectomy colonic hemorrhage. Dis Colon Rectum. 1996;39:806–10.
6. Di Giorgio P, De Luca L, Calcagno G, Rivellini G, Mandato M, De Luca B. Detachable snare versus epinephrine injection in the prevention of post-polypectomy bleeding: a randomized and controlled study. Endoscopy. 2004;36(10):860–3.
7. Choung BS, Kim SH, Ahn DS, Kwon DH, Koh KH, Sohn JY, Park WS, Kim IH, Lee SO, Lee ST, Kim SW. Incidence and risk factors of delayed post-polypectomy bleeding: a retrospective cohort study. J Clin Gastroenterol. 2014;48:784–9.
8. Repici A, Hassan C, Vitetta E, Ferrara E, Manes G, Gullotti G, Princiotta A, Dulbecco P, Gaffuri N, Bettoni E, Pagano N, Rando G, Strangio G, Carlino A, Romeo F, de Paula Pessoa Ferreira D, Zullo A, Ridola L, Malesci A. Safety of cold polypectomy for <10mm polyps at colonoscopy: a prospective multicenter study. Endoscopy. 2012;44:27–31.
9. Gimeno-Garcia AZ, de Ganzo ZA, Sosa AJ, Pérez DN, Quintero E. Incidence and predictors of post-polypectomy bleeding in colorectal polyps larger than 10 mm. Eur J Gastroenterol Hepatol. 2012;24:520–6.
10. Burgess NG, Metz AJ, Williams SJ, Singh R, Tam W, Hourigan LF, Zanati SA, Brown GJ, Sonson R, Bourke MJ. Risk factors for intra-procedural and clinically significant delayed bleeding after wide-field endoscopic mucosal resection of large colonic lesions. Clin Gastroenterol Hepatol. 2014;12:651–61.
11. Heresbach D, Kornhauser R, Seyrig JA, Coumaros D, Claviere C, Bury A, Cottereau J, Canard JM, Chaussade S, Baudet A, Casteur A, Duval O, Ponchon T, OMEGA group. A national survey of endoscopic mucosal resection for superficial gastrointestinal neoplasia. Endoscopy. 2010;42:806–13.
12. Cipolletta L, Rotondano G, Bianco MA, Buffoli F, Gizzi G, Tessari F, Italian Colorectal Endoscopic Resection (ICER) Study Group. Endoscopic resection for superficial colorectal neoplasia in Italy: a prospective multicenter study. Dig Liver Dis. 2014;46:146–51.
13. Repici A, Hassan C, De Paula Pessoa D, Pagano N, Arezzo A, Zullo A, Lorenzetti R, Marmo R. Efficacy and safety of endoscopic submucosal dissection for colorectal neoplasia: a systematic review. Endoscopy. 2012;44:137–50.

14. Fujiya M, Tanaka K, Dokoshi T, Tominaga M, Ueno N, Inaba Y, Ito T, Moriichi K, Kohgo Y. Efficacy and adverse events of EMR and endoscopic submucosal dissection for the treatment of colon neoplasms: a meta-analysis of studies comparing EMR and endoscopic submucosal dissection. Gastrointest Endosc. 2015;81(3):583e95.

15. Sawhney MS, Salfiti N, Nelson DB, Lederle FA, Bond JH. Risk factors for severe delayed post-polypectomy bleeding. Endoscopy. 2008;40:115–9.

16. Kim JH, Lee HJ, Ahn JW, Cheung DY, Kim JI, Park SH, Kim JK. Risk factors for delayed post-polypectomy hemorrhage: a case-control study. J Gastroenterol Hepatol. 2013;28:645–9.

17. Watabe H, Yamaji Y, Okamoto M, Kondo S, Ohta M, Ikenoue T, Kato J, Togo G, Matsumura M, Yoshida H, Kawabe T, Omata M. Risk assessment for delayed hemorrhagic complication of colonic polypectomy: polyp-related factors and patient related factors. Gastrointest Endosc. 2006;64:73–8.

18. Buddingh KT, Herngreen T, Haringsma J, van der Zwet WC, Vleggaar FP, Breumelhof R, Ter Borg F. Location in the right hemi-colon is an independent risk factor for delayed post-polypectomy hemorrhage: a multi-center case-control study. Am J Gastroenterol. 2011;106:1119–24.

19. Amato A, Radaelli F, Dinelli M, Crosta C, Cengia G, Beretta P, Devani M, Lochis D, Manes G, Fini L, Paggi S, Passoni GR, Repici A, SIED Lombardy group. Early and delayed complications of polypectomy in a community setting: the SPoC prospective multicentre trial. Dig Liver Dis. 2016; 48(1):43–8.

20. Dobrowolski S, Dobosz M, Babicki A, Głowacki J, Nałecz A. Blood supply of colorectal polyps correlates with risk of bleeding after colonoscopic polypectomy. Gastrointest Endosc. 2006;63:1004–9.

21. Kim HS, Kim TI, Kim WH, Kim YH, Kim HJ, Yang SK, Myung SJ, Byeon JS, Lee MS, Chung IK, Jung SA, Jeen YT, Choi JH, Choi KY, Choi H, Han DS, Song JS. Risk factors for immediate post-polypectomy bleeding of the colon: a multicenter study. Am J Gastroenterol. 2006;101:1333–41.

22. Zhang Q, Sl A, Zy C, Fu FH, Jiang B, Fc Z, Bai Y, Gong W. Assessment of risk factors for delayed colonic post-polypectomy hemorrhage: a study of 15553 polypectomies from 2005 to 2013. PLoS One. 2014;9(10):e108290.

23. Kwon MJ, Kim YS, Bae SI, Park YI, Lee KJ, Min JH, Jo SY, Kim MY, Jung HJ, Jeong SY, Yoon WJ, Kim JN, Moon JS. Risk factors for delayed post-polypectomy bleeding. Intest Res. 2015;13(2):160–5.

24. Veitch AM, Vanbiervliet G, Gershlick AH, Boustiere C, Baglin TP, Smith LA, Radaelli F, Knight E, Gralnek IM, Hassan C, Dumonceau JM. Endoscopy in patients on antiplatelet or anticoagulant therapy, including direct oral anticoagulants: British Society of Gastroenterology (BSG) and European Society of Gastrointestinal Endoscopy (ESGE) guidelines. Endoscopy. 2016;48(4):385–402.

25. Shalman D, Gerson LB. Systematic review with meta-analysis: the risk of gastrointestinal hemorrhage post-polypectomy in patients receiving anti-platelet, anti-coagulant and/or thienopyridine medications. Aliment Pharmacol Ther. 2015;42:949–56.

26. Metz AJ, Bourke MJ, Moss A, Williams SJ, Swan MP, Byth K. Factors that predict bleeding following endoscopic mucosal resection of large colonic lesions. Endoscopy. 2011;43:506–11.

27. Bahin FF, Naidoo M, Williams SJ, Hourigan LF, Ormonde DG, Raftopoulos SC, Holt BA, Sonson R, Bourke MJ. Prophylactic endoscopic coagulation to prevent bleeding after wide-field endoscopic mucosal resection of large sessile colon polyps. Clin Gastroenterol Hepatol. 2015;13:724–30.

28. Yousfi M, Gostout CJ, Baron TH, Hernandez JL, Keate R, Fleischer DE, Sorbi D. Postpolypectomy lower gastrointestinal bleeding: potential role of aspirin. Am J Gastroenterol. 2004;99:1785–9.

29. Hui AJ, Wong RM, Ching JY, Hung LC, Chung SC, Sung JJ. Risk of colonoscopic polypectomy bleeding with anticoagulants and antiplatelet agents: analysis of 1657 cases. Gastrointest Endosc. 2004;59:44–8.

30. Gandhi S, Narula N, Mosleh W, Marshall JK, Farkouh M. Meta-analysis: colonoscopic postpolypectomy bleeding in patients on continued clopidogrel therapy. Aliment Pharmacol Ther. 2013;37(10):947–52.

31. ASGE Standards of Practice Committee, Acosta RD, Abraham NS, Chandrasekhara V, Chathadi KV, Early DS, Eloubeidi MA, Evans JA, Faulx AL, Fisher DA, Fonkalsrud L, Hwang JH, Khashab MA, Lightdale JR, Muthusamy VR, Pasha SF, Saltzman JR, Shaukat A, Shergill AK, Wang A, Cash BD, JM DW. The management of antithrombotic agents for patients undergoing GI endoscopy. Gastrointest Endosc. 2016;83(1):3–16.
32. Paspatis GA, Tribonias G, Konstantinidis K, Theodoropoulou A, Vardas E, Voudoukis E, Manolaraki MM, Chainaki I, Chlouverakis G. A prospective randomized comparison of cold vs hot snare polypectomy in the occurrence of post-polypectomy bleeding in small colonic polyps. Color Dis. 2011;13(10):e345–e348. 41.
33. Ichise Y, Horiuchi A, Nakayama Y, Tanaka N. Prospective randomized comparison of cold snare polypectomy and conventional polypectomy for small colorectal polyps. Digestion. 2011;84(1):78–81.
34. Horiuchi A, Nakayama Y, Kajiyama M, Tanaka N, Sano K, Graham DY. Removal of small colorectal polyps in anticoagulated patients: a prospective randomized comparison of cold snare and conventional polypectomy. Gastrointest Endosc. 2014;79(3):417–23.
35. Monkemuller K, Neumann H, Malfertheiner P, Fry LC. Advanced colon polypectomy. Clin Gastroenterol Hepatol. 2009;7:641–52.
36. Van Gossum A, Cozzoli A, Adler M, Taton G, Cremer M. Colonoscopic snare polypectomy: analysis of 1485 resections comparing two types of current. Gastrointest Endosc. 1992;38:472–5.
37. Klein A, Bourke MJ. Advanced polypectomy and resection techniques. Gastrointest Endosc Clin N Am. 2015;25(2):303–33.
38. Burgess NG, Bahin FF, Bourke MJ. Colonic polypectomy. Gastrointest Endosc. 2015;81(4):813–35.
39. Alcaide N, Penas-Herrero I, Sancho-del-Val L, Ruiz-Zorrilla R, Barrio J, Pérez-Miranda M. Ovesco system for treatment of post-polypectomy bleeding after failure of conventional treatment. Rev Esp Enferm Dig. 2014;106:55–8.
40. Singhal S, Changela K, Papafragkakis H, Anand S, Krishnaiah M, Duddempudi S. Over the scope clip: technique and expanding clinical applications. J Clin Gastroenterol. 2013;47:749–56.
41. Fahrtash-Bahin F, Holt BA, Jayasekeran V, Williams SJ, Sonson R, Bourke MJ. Snare tip soft coagulation achieves effective and safe endoscopic hemostasis during wide-field endoscopic resection of large colonic lesions. Gastrointest Endosc. 2013;78(1):158–63.
42. Parra-Blanco A, Kaminaga N, Kojima T, Endo Y, Uragami N, Okawa N, Hattori T, Takahashi H, Fujita R. Hemoclipping for post-polypectomy and post-biopsy colonic bleeding. Gastrointest Endosc. 2000;51:37–41.
43. Slivka A, Parsons WG, Carr-Locke DL. Endoscopic band ligation for treatment of post-polypectomy hemorrhage. Gastrointest Endosc. 1994;40(2 Pt 1):230e2.
44. Burgess NG, Williams SJ, Hourigan LF, Brown GJ, Zanati SA, Singh R, Tam W, Butt J, Byth K, Bourke MJ. A management algorithm based on delayed bleeding after wide-field endoscopic mucosal resection of large colonic lesions. Clin Gastroenterol Hepatol. 2014;12(9):1525e33.
45. Terasaki M, Tanaka S, Shigita K, Asayama N, Nishiyama S, Hayashi N, Nakadoi K, Oka S, Chayama K. Risk factors for delayed bleeding after endoscopic submucosal dissection for colorectal neoplasms. Int J Color Dis. 2014;29(7):877e82.
46. Saito Y, Uraoka T, Yamaguchi Y, Hotta K, Sakamoto N, Ikematsu H, Fukuzawa M, Kobayashi N, Nasu J, Michida T, Yoshida S, Ikehara H, Otake Y, Nakajima T, Matsuda T, Saito D. A prospective, multicenter study of 1111 colorectal endoscopic submucosal dissections. Gastrointest Endosc. 2010;72(6):1217e25.
47. Pimentel-Nunes P, Dinis-Ribeiro M, Ponchon T, Repici A, Vieth M, De Ceglie A, Amato A, Berr F, Bhandari P, Bialek A, Conio M, Haringsma J, Langner C, Meisner S, Messmann H, Morino M, Neuhaus H, Piessevaux H, Rugge M, Saunders BP, Robaszkiewicz M, Seewald S, Kashin S, Dumonceau JM, Hassan C, Deprez PH. Endoscopic submucosal dissection: European Society of Gastrointestinal Endoscopy (ESGE) guideline. Endoscopy. 2015;47(9):829e54.

48. Lee SH, Chung IK, Kim SJ, Kim JO, Ko BM, Kim WH, Kim HS, Park DI, Kim HJ, Byeon JS, Yang SK, Jang BI, Jung SA, Jeen YT, Choi JH, Choi H, Han DS, Song JS. Comparison of post-polypectomy bleeding between epinephrine and saline submucosal injection for large colon polyps by conventional polypectomy: a prospective randomized, multicenter study. World J Gastroenterol. 2007;13:2973–7.
49. Dobrowolski S, Dobosz M, Babicki A, Dymecki D, Hać S. Prophylactic submucosal saline-adrenaline injection in colonoscopic polypectomy: prospective randomized study. Surg Endosc. 2004;18:990–3.
50. Facciorusso A, Di Maso M, Antonino M, Del Prete V, Panella C, Barone M, Muscatiello N. Polidocanol injection decreases the bleeding rate after colon polypectomy: a propensity score analysis. Gastrointest Endosc. 2015;82(2):350–8.
51. Shioji K, Suzuki Y, Kobayashi M, Nakamura A, Azumaya M, Takeuchi M, Baba Y, Honma T, Narisawa R. Prophylactic clip application does not decrease delayed bleeding after colono-scopic polypectomy. Gastrointest Endosc. 2003;57:691–4.
52. Liaquat H, Rohn E, Rex DK. Prophylactic clip closure reduced the risk of delayed post-polypectomy hemorrhage: experience in 277 clipped large sessile or flat colorectal lesions and 247 control lesions. Gastrointest Endosc. 2013;77:401–7.
53. Li LY, Liu QS, Li L, Cao YJ, Yuan Q, Liang SW, Qu CM. A meta-analysis and systematic review of prophylactic endoscopic treatments for post-polypectomy bleeding. Int J Color Dis. 2011;26:709–19.
54. Lee CK, Lee SH, Park JY, Lee TH, Chung IK, Park SH, Kim HS, Kim SJ. Prophylactic argon plasma coagulation ablation does not decrease delayed post-polypectomy bleeding. Gastrointest Endosc. 2009;70:353–61.
55. Park CH, Jung YS, Nam E, Eun CS, Park DI, Han DS. Comparison of efficacy of prophylactic endoscopic therapies for postpolypectomy bleeding in the colorectum: a systematic review and network meta-analysis. Am J Gastroenterol. 2016;111(9):1230–43. Li lylee ck
56. Sethi A, Song LM. Adverse events related to colonic endoscopic mucosal resection and polyp-ectomy. Gastrointest Endosc Clin N Am. 2015;25(1):55–69.
57. Thirumurthi S, Raju GS. Management of polypectomy complications. Gastrointest Endosc Clin N Am. 2015;25(2):335–57.
58. Levy I, Gralnek IM. Complications of diagnostic colonoscopy, upper endoscopy, and enteros-copy. Best Pract Res Clin Gastroenterol. 2016;30(5):705–18.
59. Ma MX, Bourke MJ. Complications of endoscopic polypectomy, endoscopic mucosal resec-tion and endoscopic submucosal dissection in the colon. Best Pract Res Clin Gastroenterol. 2016;30(5):749–67.
60. Broeders E, Al-Taher M, Peeters K, Bouvy N. Verres needle desufflation as an effective treat-ment option for colonic perforation after colonoscopy. Surg Laparosc Endosc Percutan Tech. 2015;25(2):e61–4.
61. Tutticci N, Bourke MJ. Advanced endoscopic resection in the colon: recent innovations, cur-rent limitations and future directions. Expert Rev Gastroenterol Hepatol. 2014;8(2):161–77.
62. Wada Y, Kudo SE, Tanaka S, Saito Y, Iishii H, Ikematsu H, Igarashi M, Saitoh Y, Inoue Y, Kobayashi K, Hisabe T, Tsuruta O, Kashida H, Ishikawa H, Sugihara K. Predictive factors for complications in endoscopic resection of large colorectal lesions: a multicenter prospective study. Surg Endosc. 2015;29(5):1216–22.
63. Kim ES, Cho KB, Park KS, Lee KI, Jang BK, Chung WJ, Hwang JS. Factors predictive of perforation during endoscopic submucosal dissection for the treatment of colorectal tumors. Endoscopy. 2011;43:573–8.
64. Iqbal CW, Cullinane DC, Schiller HJ, Sawyer MD, Zietlow SP, Farley DR. Surgical manage-ment and outcomes of 165 colonoscopic perforations from a single institution. Arch Surg. 2008;143:701–6.
65. Raju GS. Gastrointestinal perforations: role of endoscopic closure. Curr Opin Gastroenterol. 2011;27:418–22.
66. Oka S, Tanaka S, Kanao H, et al. Current status in the occurrence of postoperative bleeding, perforation and residual/local recurrence during colonoscopic treatment in Japan. Dig Endosc. 2010;22:376–80.

67. Raju GS, Saito Y, Matsuda T, Kaltenbach T, Soetikno R. Endoscopic management of colonoscopic perforations (with videos). Gastrointest Endosc. 2011;74:1380–8.
68. Bielawska B, Day AG, Lieberman DA, Hookey LC. Risk factors for early colonoscopic perforation include non-gastroenterologist endoscopists: a multivariable analysis. Clin Gastroenterol Hepatol. 2014;12:85–92.
69. Buchner AM, Guarner-Argente C, Ginsberg GG. Outcomes of EMR of defiant colorectal lesions directed to an endoscopy referral center. Gastrointest Endosc. 2012;76:255–63.
70. Seo EH, Kim TO, Park MJ, Joo HR, Heo NY, Park J, Park SH, Yang SY, Moon YS. Optimal preparation-to-colonoscopy interval in split-dose PEG bowel preparation determines satisfactory bowel preparation quality: an observational prospective study. Gastrointest Endosc. 2012;75(3):583–90.
71. Pissas D, Ypsilantis E, Papagrigoriadis S, Hayee B, Haji A. Endoscopic management of iatrogenic perforations during endoscopic mucosal resection (EMR) and endoscopic submucosal dissection (ESD) for colorectal polyps: a case series. Therap Adv Gastroenterol. 2015;8(4):176–81.
72. Rex DK. Water filling and carbon dioxide insufflation: tools for every colonoscopist. Clin Gastroenterol Hepatol. 2015;13(11):1981–3.
73. ASGE Technology Committee, Maple JT, Abu Dayyeh BK, Chauhan SS, Hwang JH, Komanduri S, Manfredi M, Konda V, Murad FM, Siddiqui UD, Banerjee S. Endoscopic submucosal dissection. Gastrointest Endosc. 2015;81(6):1311–25.
74. Holt BA, Jayasekeran V, Sonson R, Bourke MJ. Topical submucosal chromoendoscopy defines the level of resection in colonic EMR and may improve procedural safety (with video). Gastrointest Endosc. 2013;77:949–53.
75. Swan MP, Bourke MJ, Moss A, Williams SJ, Hopper A, Metz A. The target sign: an endoscopic marker for the resection of the muscularis propria and potential perforation during colonic endoscopic mucosal resection. Gastrointest Endosc. 2011;73:79–85.
76. Tang SJ. Zipper clip closure of colonoscopic perforations. Gastrointest Endosc. 2017;85(4):867–9.
77. Kobara H, Mori H, Fujihara S, Nishiyama N, Chiyo T, Yamada T, Fujiwara M, Okano K, Suzuki Y, Murota M, Ikeda Y, Oryu M, Abo Ellail M, Masaki T. Outcomes of gastrointestinal defect closure with an over-the-scope clip system in a multicenter experience: an analysis of a successful suction method. World J Gastroenterol. 2017;23(9):1645–56.
78. Honegger C, Valli PV, Wiegand N, Bauerfeind P, Gubler C. Establishment of over-the-scope-clips (OTSC®) in daily endoscopic routine. United European Gastroenterol J. 2017;5(2):247–54.
79. Weiland T, Fehlker M, Gottwald T, Schurr MO. Performance of the OTSC system in the endoscopic closure of iatrogenic gastrointestinal perforations: a systematic review. Surg Endosc. 2013;27:2258–74.
80. Paraskeva KD, Paspatis GA. Management of bleeding and perforation after colonoscopy. Expert Rev Gastroenterol Hepatol. 2014;8(8):963–72.
81. Kantsevoy SV, Bitner M, Mitrakov AA, Thuluvath PJ. Endoscopic suturing closure of large mucosal defects after endoscopic submucosal dissection is technically feasible, fast, and eliminates the need for hospitalization. Gastrointest Endosc. 2014;79:503–7.
82. Cho SB, Lee WS, Joo YE, Kim HR, Park SW, Park CH, Kim HS, Choi SK, Rew JS. Therapeutic options for iatrogenic colon perforation: feasibility of endoscopic clip closure and predictors of the need for early surgery. Surg Endosc. 2012;26:473–9.
83. Kim JS, Kim BW, Kim JI, Kim JH, Kim SW, Ji JS, Lee BI, Choi H. Endoscopic clip closure versus surgery for the treatment of iatrogenic colon perforations developed during diagnostic colonoscopy: a review of 115,285 patients. Surg Endosc. 2013;27:501–4.
84. Jehangir A, Bennett KM, Rettew AC, Fadahunsi O, Shaikh B, Donato A. Post-polypectomy electrocoagulation syndrome: a rare cause of acute abdominal pain. J Community Hosp Intern Med Perspect. 2015;5(5):29147.
85. Cha JM, Lim KS, Lee SH, Joo YE, Hong SP, Kim TI, Kim HG, Park DI, Kim SE, Yang DH, Shin JE. Clinical outcomes and risk factors of postpolypectomy coagulation syndrome: a multicenter, retrospective, case-control study. Endoscopy. 2013;45:202–7.

Anticoagulants and Antiplatelet Agents in Patients Undergoing Polypectomy

9

Angelo Milano, Francesco Laterza, Konstantinos Efthymakis, Antonella Bonitatibus, and Matteo Neri

9.1 Introduction

Antithrombotic drugs are frequently used to reduce thromboembolic risk in conditions such as atrial fibrillation (AF), coronary heart disease (CHD), venous thromboembolism (VTE), and endoprostheses. These are classified in two categories: anticoagulants (ACs) and antiplatelet agents (APA). The first act on the clotting cascade, while the latter impede platelet aggregation. The ACs include (1) vitamin K antagonists (e.g., warfarin), (2) heparin derivatives (e.g., unfractionated heparin (UFH) and low molecular weight heparin (LMWH), fondaparinux, e.g., Arixtra), and (3) direct oral anticoagulants (DOAC) that include direct factor Xa inhibitors, like rivaroxaban (Xarelto) and apixaban (Eliquis), as well as dabigatran (Pradaxa), a direct thrombin inhibitor. APA span from classical agents such as aspirin to the newer thienopyridine class that includes clopidogrel and prasugrel and the most recent cyclopentyl triazolo-pyrimidines, like ticagrelor. Platelet aggregation inhibitors are frequently used in association, unlike anticoagulants that are typically used in monotherapy, in order to reduce thromboembolic risk in patients presenting with a variety of predisposing conditions, by ultimately impeding clot formation.

Consequently, major adverse events of such treatments include GI bleeding, and their use increases the risk of hemorrhage, especially in case of endoscopic interventions [1–3]. This is particularly true for anticoagulants and all the more for the newer DOAC, which seem to increase bleeding risk when compared to warfarin and for which, up to now, a reversal agent is not available even though some are in development. For this reason, when endoscopic procedures are necessary, both bleeding

A. Milano • F. Laterza • K. Efthymakis • A. Bonitatibus • M. Neri (✉)
Department of Medicine and Ageing Sciences and Center for Excellence on Ageing
and Translational Medicine (CeSI-MeT), "G. D'Annunzio" University and Foundation,
Chieti, Italy

Digestive Endoscopy Unit, SS. Annunziata Hospital, Chieti, Italy
e-mail: matteo.neri@unich.it

© Springer International Publishing AG 2018
A. Facciorusso, N. Muscatiello (eds.), *Colon Polypectomy*,
https://doi.org/10.1007/978-3-319-59457-6_9

121

and thrombotic risks should be considered. In fact, bleeding risk associated to prescribed antithrombotic regimen (e.g., aspirin, clopidogrel, prasugrel, DOAC) and
thrombotic risk in case of drug interruption need careful balancing, based on predisposing condition to thrombosis (low-risk versus high-risk condition) and bleeding
risk inherent to the endoscopic procedure (low-risk versus high-risk procedure).
Lastly, in some cases, reevaluation may be important in determining the appropri-
ateness of prescribed treatments according to current indications (e.g., ASA in
primary prophylaxis).

Polypectomy, endoscopic mucosal resection (EMR), and submucosal dissection
(ESD) are included among the high bleeding risk procedures in drug-free patients;
when considering treated subjects, appropriate evaluation of anticoagulant or antithrombotic regimens is fundamental for cost-effective management, tailored to the
individual patient.

9.2   Procedure-Related Bleeding Risk

An exhaustive literature discussion on bleeding risk in patients undergoing mucosal
resection during colonoscopy is difficult mainly due to differences in study design,
endoscopic techniques considered, and, more importantly, the broad definitions
used. Crucially, the latter can result in rather heterogeneous events being grouped
under the same term, when a more precise classification could prove useful in
assessing "real-life" GI bleeding risk and hence guide periprocedural management.
For instance, polypectomy-related hemorrhage can refer either to procedural bleeding (PB), which may occur during procedures and can be self-limiting or controlled
by hemostatic techniques, or post-procedural bleeding (PPB), which can be self-
limiting or requiring an unplanned hospital admission, blood transfusions, and/or
repeated endoscopic hemostatic procedures [4]. These important distinctions are
sometimes not taken into account in published studies, resulting in confusing and
not comparable results. Moreover, most studies are retrospective in nature, with low
event prevalence ranging from 0.6 to 2.2% in sample sizes of >1000 cases [5–12].
In one recent study [12], mean time of delayed onset of the bleeding was
4.0 ± 2.9 days, in line with previous data [5]. The most important factor predisposing to bleeding was polyp size, with a 9% increased risk (OR 1.09; 95% CI, 1.0–1.2)
for every millimeter of increase in polyp diameter [5]. Moreover, the use of a non-
controlled cutting current and use of pure cutting current are also independent risk
factors for PPB [13, 14]. In the case of EMR, bleeding risk seems to be higher than
polypectomy, with an incidence of immediate bleeding between 3.7 and 11.3% and
of delayed bleeding between 0.6 and 6.2% [15, 16]. Nevertheless, for lesions
<10 mm, EMR is comparable to polypectomy. Compared to the previous proce-
dures, ESD seems to show a higher bleeding rate, with an OD of 2.20 (95% CI,
1.58–3.07) [17]. In two studies on colonic polypectomy (polyp size <1 cm) in
patients assuming warfarin, the authors found that hemorrhages requiring blood
transfusion happened in 0.8% of the cases, despite prophylactic clips were applied
routinely [18] and that cold snare resection compared to hot snare resection showed

minor immediate hemorrhage (5.7 vs 23%) or delayed hemorrhage (0 vs 14%) [19]. Unfortunately, data on patient bleeding risk in each study are lacking, so that these percentages may not reflect outcomes in specific clinical scenarios.

9.3   Polypectomy and Warfarin

In 2016, managing guidelines for patients under antithrombotic treatment undergoing endoscopic procedures have been revised both by the ASGE and jointly by the ESGE and BSG [4, 20], with some notable differences. The American guidelines stratify risk for thromboembolic events in anticoagulated patients in three categories (high, medium, and low; see Table 9.1). On the contrary, in the joint European guidelines, only two categories are considered (high and low risk), in order to better discriminate, in case of warfarin discontinuation, which patient will benefit from a bridging treatment with low molecular weight heparin (LMWH) and who will not (see Table 9.2). For example, one should note the differences in approach for patients with atrial fibrillation (AF), with or without valvular disease. The latter group in fact, based on a study conducted on 1884 patients, is considered at low risk

Table 9.1 Risk of thromboembolism in patients on anticoagulation [20]

Annual risk	Mechanical heart valve	History of VTE or thrombophilic conditions
High	Any mitral valve prosthesis Any caged-ball or tilting disc aortic valve prosthesis Recent (within 6 months) CVA or TIA	Recent (within 3 months) VTE Severe thrombophilia (deficiency of protein C, protein S, or antithrombin; antiphospholipid antibodies; multiple abnormalities)
Medium	Bileaflet aortic valve prosthesis and one or more of the following risk factors: AF, prior CVA or TIA, hypertension, diabetes, congestive heart failure, age >75 years	VTE within the past 3–12 months Non-severe thrombophilia (heterozygous factor V Leiden or prothrombin gene mutation) Recurrent VTE Active cancer (treated within 6 months or palliative)
Low	Bileaflet aortic valve prosthesis without AF and no other risk factors for CVA	VTE >12 months previous and no other risk factors

Table 9.2 Risk stratification of patients on warfarin therapy. Bridging treatment with LMWH during warfarin discontinuation benefits high-risk conditions [4]

Low-risk condition	High-risk condition
• Prosthetic metal heart valve in aortic position • Xenograft heart valve • AF without valvular disease • >3 months after VTE • Thrombophilia syndromes (liaise with hematologist)	• Prosthetic metal heart valve in mitral position • Prosthetic heart valve and AF • AF and mitral stenosis • <3 months after VTE

for thrombotic complications and therefore does not require bridging therapy with heparin [21]. In this study, patients were randomized to bridge therapy with LMWH versus placebo. While there were no differences in incidence of arterial thromboembolism (0.3% vs 0.4%, respectively), an increased incidence of bleeding in the heparin group was observed (3.2% vs 1.3%, respectively). The ASGE guidelines, on the contrary, consider AF without valvular disease as a more complex scenario. They, in fact, suggest the use of the CHA_2DS_2-VASc score to evaluate thromboembolic risk in a case-by-case manner [22]. This score includes different thromboembolic risk factors, including congestive heart failure, hypertension, older age, diabetes, stroke, prior myocardial infarction (MI) or peripheral artery disease, or aortic plaque and sex. The higher the score (ranging from 1 to 9), the greater the thromboembolic risk. A score of ≥ 2 identifies patients at high risk, suggesting bridging therapy in case of warfarin interruption.

In summary, regarding patients on warfarin but with a low risk for thrombotic events, indications dictate warfarin discontinuation 5 days before polypectomy and a confirmed INR value of <1.5 prior to the procedure. After the procedure, warfarin can be restarted on the same day. In the case of patients at high risk for thromboembolism, warfarin should be managed as above, but adding bridging therapy with LMWH is recommended. In particular, LMWH treatment should start 2 days after warfarin discontinuation and should be stopped 24 h prior to the procedure, in order to minimize the risk of bleeding. The day after the procedure, LMWH should be restarted until a therapeutic INR under warfarin is achieved. Although the above treatment management should minimize both bleeding and thrombotic complications in the majority of patients, consultation with a cardiologist may be desirable in particular cases and clinical scenarios.

9.4   Direct Oral Anticoagulants

DOAC have been widely prescribed since their approval, thanks to their advantages when compared to vitamin K antagonists. While both can be assumed orally, DOAC do not need blood sampling to evaluate efficacy, have a fixed dose, and show minor interaction with other drugs and not at all with food, when compared to warfarin. As with other anticoagulants, in case of high-risk endoscopic procedures, it is important to balance bleeding risks due to intensity of anticoagulation with thromboembolic risks linked to the patient's condition. DOAC are approved for the prevention and treatment of deep vein thrombosis and pulmonary embolism and the prevention of stroke or embolus in patients with non-rheumatic atrial fibrillation, as such patients in DOAC treatment are considered at low risk of thromboembolism. For this reason, it could be inferred that there is no need for bridging therapy with LMWH in this patients. This was confirmed by observational data which show that bridging therapy in case of DOAC interruption not only does not reduce the incidence of cardiovascular or thromboembolic events, but appears to be associated with an increased incidence of major bleeding events (6.5 vs 1.8%; $p < 0.001$) [23].

The pharmacodynamic effects of DOAC depend obviously on their pharmacokinetic profile and their blood accumulation. Unfortunately, monitoring treatments is difficult as tests such as PT or APTT can only indicate the gross level of anticoagulation (supratherapeutic, therapeutic or subtherapeutic); plasma concentrations of most DOAC cannot be determined in a clinical setting. Moreover, test results are heavily influenced by dose-timing and other factors that influence pharmacokinetics. In the case of dabigatran, Hemoclot®, a thrombin inhibitor assay, can be used to determine drug concentration [24]. Anti-factor Xa assays are sensitive to specific factor Xa inhibitors and require specific calibrators and controls; the anti-factor Xa chromogenic method can be used for plasma concentration determination of Xa inhibitors in standard therapeutic doses [25, 26].

While readily accessible inexpensive tests are currently unavailable, it should be kept in mind that all DOAC are mainly excreted in the urine, and therefore renal function is an important limiting factor for their blood accumulation, particularly for dabigatran. The half-life of dabigatran, in fact, can vary from 12 to 13 h, for a creatinine clearance (CrCL) of 80 mL/min, to 27 h should CrCl fall to <30 mL/min. Because of this dabigatran should not be used in case of a CrCl of ≤30 mL/min; a reduced dose, from 150 to 110 mg bid, should be prescribed if CrCL is <50 mL/min or in patients over 80 years of age. While no liver toxicity has been observed for dabigatran, it can be prescribed in case of liver disease without coagulopathy. Rivaroxaban has a half-life that may vary from 7 to 11 h. It is mainly metabolized by the liver (about 65%), but it can also be equally prescribed in case of liver disease without coagulopathy. Considering its renal clearance, no accumulation of the drug has been observed down to a CrCl of 15 mL/min, below which the drug should not be administered. Nevertheless, a dose reduction from 20 to 15 mg od is recommended if CrCl is between 15 and 30 mL/min. Similar recommendations are in effect for apixaban and edoxaban, both of which have less than 50% of the kidney clearance [4].

In terms of safety, unavailability of an antagonist is the primary limiting factor for DOAC use. Recently, some antidotes have been studied in animal models with encouraging results; in 2015 idarucizumab (Praxbind) was the first antidote for dabigatran approved by the FDA for use in patients with life-threatening conditions [27]. Regarding gastrointestinal (GI) bleeding risk in patients under DOAC, current data seem to support a better safety profile than previously described. In fact, while initial studies showed an increased risk of GI bleeding [28, 29] compared to warfarin, other studies have produced opposite results [30]. Previous publications stressed the good safety profile of DOAC in terms of major bleeding or intracranial bleeding when compared with warfarin. On the contrary, high-dose DOAC were associated with a significant increase in GI bleeding risk [31]. A recent study [32] published in 2017 conducted on a population of about 7000 patients in "real life" (mean age 70 years) has showed that patients on warfarin have an increased risk of GI bleeding when compared with those on dabigatran, rivaroxaban, and apixaban, with an OR of 4.13 (95% CI, 1.69–10.09). A study published by Abraham et al. [33] directly assessed the GI safety profiles of dabigatran, rivaroxaban, and apixaban in a population of 43,300 patients. In terms of gastrointestinal bleeding risk, the authors

observed that apixaban showed the best safety profile among the three, while rivaroxaban displayed the worst. Moreover, while GI bleeding risk is known to increase
with age, apixaban preserved its safety profile in older patients.

9.5   DOAC and Polypectomy

Considering the importance of renal function for the pharmacodynamics of DOAC,
their management prior to high-risk endoscopic procedures (polypectomy, EMR, ESD)
should include blood sampling for the evaluation of CrCl, mainly in older subjects or
severe kidney pathology. Counseling with a hematologist should be considered in case
of a rapid reduction in renal function. In general, DOAC should be discontinued at least
48 h prior to endoscopy (detailed discontinuation times according to CrCl are summarized in the Tables 9.3, 9.4, and 9.5). In terms of drug resumption after endoscopy, it is
important to summarize some notable differences between DOAC and warfarin: while
it takes several days to restore normal coagulation after warfarin discontinuation, only
3–4 h are generally needed for the anticoagulant effect of DOAC to be reversed. Owing

Table 9.3 Periprocedural management of dabigatran (Pradaxa) [34]

Creatinine clearance (mL/min)	Time to onset of action (h)	Half-life (h)	Timing of discontinuation before procedure (days)
>80	1.25–3	13 (11–22)	2–3
50–80	1.25–3	15 (12–34)	2–3
30–49	1.25–3	18 (13–33)	3–4
≤29	1.25–3	27 (22–25)	4–6

Table 9.4 Periprocedural management of apixaban (Eliquis) [35]

Creatinine clearance (mL/min)	Time to onset of action (h)	Timing of discontinuation before procedure (days)
>60	1–3	1–2
30–59	1–3	3
15–29	1–3	4

Table 9.5 Periprocedural management of rivaroxaban (Xarelto) [35]

Creatinine clearance (mL/min)	Time to onset of action (h)	Timing of discontinuation before procedure (days)
>90	2–4	1–2
60–90	2–4	2
30–59	2–4	3
15–29	2–4	4

Table 9.6 DOAC and high-risk endoscopic procedures [4]

High-risk procedure		
Warfarin		DOAC

Low-risk condition	High-risk condition	Low-risk condition
• Prosthetic metal heart valve in aortic position	• Prosthetic metal heart valve in mitral position	High-risk condition
• Xenograft heart valve	• Prosthetic heart valve	
• AF without valvular disease >3 months after VTE	• and AF	
• Thrombophilia syndromes (liaise with hematologist)	• AF and mitral stenosis	
	• <3 months after VTE	

Stop warfarin 5 days before endoscopy	Stop warfarin 5 days before endoscopy	Take last dose of drug ≥48 h before procedure
• Check INR prior to procedure to ensure INR <1.5	• Start LMWH 2 days after stopping warfarin	• Consult individual drug tables according to renal function
• Restart warfarin evening of procedure with usual daily dose	• Give last dose of LMWH ≥24 h before procedure	• In case of deteriorating renal function liaise with hematologist
• Check INR 1 week later to ensure adequate anticoagulation	• Restart warfarin evening of procedure with usual dose	
	• Continue LMWH until INR adequate	

to this and the fact that there are insufficient data to define optimal timings for DOAC resumption, current guidelines on this topic suggest reintroduction of these drugs as soon as possible. Because of their short onset of action, if a DOAC cannot be reintroduced within 24 h after a high-risk procedure (e.g., in case of concerns regarding adequate hemostasis), then thromboprophylaxis with bridging therapies should be considered for patients at high risk for thromboembolism.

The management of DOAC during polypectomy, EMR, and ESD is summarized in Table 9.6.

9.6 Antiplatelet Agents (APA)

Platelets are activated by multiple agonists through numerous intracellular second messenger pathways and complex networks. Platelet activation results in their adhesion and aggregation at sites of vascular injury. In addition, a major role of platelets in coagulation is to provide an anionic phospholipidic surface for the assembly of the macromolecular coagulation factor complexes required for the generation of thrombin and subsequent clot formation. APA are able to inhibit platelet activation by blocking specific membrane receptors of thrombocytes, responsible for intracellular second messenger activation; these include receptors for thrombin, adenosine diphosphate (ADP), collagen, thromboxane, and epinephrine [36].

9.7   Aspirin

Aspirin (acetylsalicylic acid, ASA), a time-honored antiplatelet agent, is an irreversible nonselective cyclooxygenase (COX) inhibitor. It is used alone or, in patients with coronary stents, in combination with other APA to prevent stent thrombosis [37]. Platelets synthesize thromboxane in response to specific agonists; its receptor is present on the cytoplasmic membrane of platelets and other tissues. Thromboxane synthesis is dependent on COX; aspirin irreversible inhibits COX activity by acetylation. In fact, although the half-life of aspirin is approximately 20 min, its pharmacodynamic effect persists for the duration of the platelet lifespan (7–10 days), as platelets are unable to replenish COX enzymatic activity by synthesis.

9.8   Thienopyridines

Thienopyridines function by inhibiting ADP-induced platelet aggregation. *Ticlopidine*, a first-generation thienopyridine agent previously used in dual antiplatelet regimens, has largely been supplanted in clinical use by newer agents, mainly because of its hematologic side effects. *Clopidogrel*, the main drug in this category, is a prodrug that requires hepatic metabolism for activation through the CYP2C19 pathway. It is used in the treatment of recent acute coronary syndromes, such as unstable angina, myocardial infarction (MI), recent stroke, or established peripheral arterial disease [38]. It is a more potent antiplatelet agent compared to aspirin, with which it has an established synergistic effect. Both drugs are frequently used in association (dual antiplatelet therapy, DAPT), although combination therapy increases bleeding risk, especially in patients undergoing high-risk endoscopic procedures. Similarly to aspirin, the antiplatelet action of clopidogrel is irreversible, and platelet function has been demonstrated to return to normal within 5–7 days of withdrawal, based on the regenerative production of clopidogrel-naive platelets [39, 40]. *Prasugrel* is a new thienopyridine. Like clopidogrel, it is a prodrug and requires hepatic metabolism for activation; however, activation pathways differ, as prasugrel is converted by CYP3A4 and CYP2B6 [41]. It is also a nonreversible platelet aggregation inhibitor and should be withheld for 7 days before an elective high-risk procedure.

9.9   Cyclopentyl Triazolo-Pyrimidines

Cyclopentyl triazolo-pyrimidines (CPTP) are a new class of antiplatelet agents, mainly represented by *ticagrelor*, a direct-acting reversible inhibitor of the ADP receptor P2Y12. Similarly to prasugrel, it is metabolized by the CYP3A4 cytochrome; however, it is not a prodrug, as both the parent drug and its metabolite are active antiplatelet agents. It is mainly used in the treatment of acute coronary syndrome with or without coronary stents. Compared to clopidogrel and prasugrel, ticagrelor has both a more rapidly established and a more pronounced inhibitory

Table 9.7 APA and duration of action [20]

Agent (class)	Duration of action
Aspirin (ASA)	7–10 days
NSAIDs	Varies
Clopidogrel (thienopyridines)	5–7 days
Prasugrel (thienopyridines)	5–7 days
Ticlopidine (thienopyridines)	10–14 days
Ticagrelor (cyclopentyl triazolo-pyrimidines)	3–5 days

effect on platelet aggregation [2]. Because of its rapid onset and offset, its effects on platelet inhibition decline rapidly over a 72-h period after cessation, and platelet activity is near normal at 5 days [42].

APA and relative duration of action are summarized in Table 9.7.

9.10   APA and Post-Procedural Bleeding

In patients undergoing antithrombotic and anticoagulant therapy, polypectomy, endoscopic mucosal resection (EMR), and endoscopic submucosal dissection (ESD) are elective endoscopic procedures classified as high-risk procedures for bleeding by the British Society of Gastroenterology (BSG), the European Society of Gastrointestinal Endoscopy (ESGE), and the American Society for Gastrointestinal Endoscopy (ASGE). However, from a cardiovascular point of view, these patients are considered at high and low risk for thrombotic events on the basis of their underlying medical conditions and prior surgery or prosthesis [20, 36]. Therefore, adequate management of APA before elective endoscopy relies on a balanced evaluation of both procedure-related bleeding risks and patient-related risk for thrombosis [43]. The probability of a thromboembolic event related to a temporary drug interruption depends on the specific indication for antithrombotic therapy and individual patient characteristics. High-risk scenarios for thrombosis in patients on APA include recent placement of drug-eluting coronary stents ($\leq$12 months) or bare metal coronary stents ($\leq$1 month); acute coronary syndrome (ACS) and bare metal coronary stenting 12 months prior to endoscopy are also considered at high risk for thrombosis [20, 44]. Endoscopists should pay attention to specific clinical risk factors that predispose to higher rates of stent occlusion beyond the first year after stent insertion, as modifications of antiplatelet regimens must be done cautiously in such cases. Late stent thrombosis occurs an average rate of 0.6% per year over the first 3 years after implantation [45]. Approximately one in five patients with a prior history of stent occlusion will experience a second event, with a cumulative risk of cardiac death of 27.9%. Furthermore, patients affected by ACS or ST elevation MI, diabetes, renal failure, diffuse coronary artery disease, or with a history of multivessel percutaneous coronary intervention are also at higher risk of stent occlusion or ACS events after suspension of antithrombotic therapy [46].

Considering antiplatelet agents, aspirin monotherapy has been found to be safe in colonoscopic polypectomy [36, 47]. It is true also that studies on patients receiving ASA in the context of endoscopic submucosal dissection (ESD) or large (>20 mm) colonic endoscopic mucosal resections (EMR) have found an increased risk of hemorrhage [13, 36, 48, 49]. However, thrombotic risks should also be considered particularly in patients receiving aspirin for secondary prevention, as they are at greater risk from discontinuation of therapy than those taking it for primary prevention: in patients on long-term low-dose aspirin for secondary prevention, aspirin interruption is associated with a threefold increased risk of cardiovascular or cerebrovascular events, 70% of which occur within 7–10 days after interruption [50]. On the other hand, hemorrhage secondary to high-risk endoscopic procedures can often be controlled by endoscopic therapeutic procedures, and it is rarely fatal, while a thrombotic stroke may result in lifelong disability, and a major cardiac event may result in death. Balancing thromboembolic and bleeding risks is crucial and ultimately needs to be assessed on an individual patient basis, with special caution when discontinuing aspirin prescribed for secondary prevention of ischemic or thrombotic events [4].

Concerning clopidogrel, available data are controversial as treatment discontinuation is the dominant risk factor for coronary artery stent thrombosis in patients with drug-eluting stents, with events occurring as early as 5–10 days after cessation of clopidogrel therapy [51]. Owing to this fact, only 48% of respondents discontinued clopidogrel before a colonoscopic polypectomy, as shown by a survey of gastroenterologists in the USA [52]. In 2013, a meta-analysis assessing the real risk of post-procedural bleeding (PPB) related to clopidogrel was performed and integrated in the current ESGE guidelines. Although in this meta-analysis polyp size was less than 10 mm in 88% of total cases, and the proportion of patients on DAPT ranged from 54 to 87.8%, the authors found a significantly increased overall risk of delayed PPB (RR = 4.66; 95% CI, 2.37–9.17) [53]. No data on PPB in patients taking prasugrel or ticagrelor were available [4].

The impact of APA on colonic post-EMR bleeding was evaluated in two recent prospective observational studies and one randomized control trial comparing endoscopic prophylactic coagulation of visible vessels compared to no prophylaxis for wide-field EMR (>2 cm). These studies showed that clinically significant post-EMR bleeding was associated to the use of aspirin; no conclusions were drawn for clopidogrel-associated bleeding risk as only 20 patients were on such treatment. No data are available regarding the management of prasugrel or ticagrelor in relation to colonic EMR [13, 49]. Regarding post-ESD bleeding, insufficient data are available on the role of aspirin or clopidogrel alone. Two studies have reported no association between post-ESD bleeding in patients on antithrombotic agents, but the drugs were discontinued 1 week prior to the procedure [54, 55]. No data are available regarding treatment with prasugrel or ticagrelor in this context [4].

Concerning dual APA therapy, a review of 161 reported cases of late stent thrombosis (>30 days but <1 year after stent placement) and very late stent thrombosis (>1 year after stent placement) shows that patients who discontinued both ASA and thienopyridine had a median time to event of 7 days; in those who discontinued

Table 9.8 APA and high-risk endoscopic procedures [4]

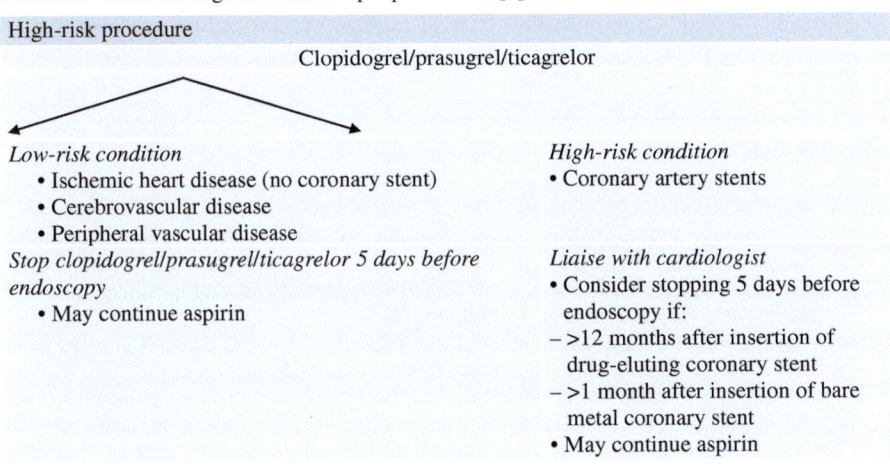

High-risk procedure

Clopidogrel/prasugrel/ticagrelor

Low-risk condition	*High-risk condition*
• Ischemic heart disease (no coronary stent) • Cerebrovascular disease • Peripheral vascular disease	• Coronary artery stents
Stop clopidogrel/prasugrel/ticagrelor 5 days before endoscopy • May continue aspirin	*Liaise with cardiologist* • Consider stopping 5 days before endoscopy if: – >12 months after insertion of drug-eluting coronary stent – >1 month after insertion of bare metal coronary stent • May continue aspirin

thienopyridine but remained on ASA, the median time to an event was 122 days. A total of six cases (6%) of stent thrombosis within 10 days of thienopyridine cessation was reported, suggesting that short-term discontinuation between 30 days and 1 year from drug-eluting coronary stent placement might be relatively safe [51]. For this reasons, the American College of Cardiology Foundation and American College of Gastroenterology consensus statement suggests that in patients receiving DAPT, only clopidogrel should be stopped 5 days before polypectomy when thrombotic risk is low, while a cardiologic consultation is needed for high-risk patients. In case of a very high thrombotic risk (e.g., within 30 days after coronary stent placement), any elective endoscopic procedures should be postponed. Clopidogrel should be resumed after the procedure, once hemostasis has been confirmed during endoscopy.

The management of APA and DAPT during polypectomy, EMR, and ESD is summarized in Table 9.8.

Conclusion

Platelet aggregation inhibitors and anticoagulants can increase the risk of hemorrhage in patients undergoing endoscopic interventions, particularly in high-risk procedures such as polypectomy, endoscopic mucosal resections, and submucosal dissection. Newer agents (DOAC) seem to further increase bleeding risk when compared to warfarin; furthermore, they currently lack reversal agents and need to be managed based on pharmacokinetic profiles and renal function. However, bleeding risk during endoscopic procedures needs to be balanced with the actual thrombotic risk of the individual patient, particularly considering that procedure-related hemorrhage can often be prevented or controlled by current prophylactic and therapeutic techniques and is rarely fatal, while thrombotic events are unpredictable and difficult to resolve and are associated to high rates of hospitalization, disability, and death. Careful evaluation of the individual patient and treatment discontinuation or bridging according to the underlying thromboembolic risk status and type of endoscopic procedure are warranted in order to maximize cost-effectiveness and safety.

References

1. Abraham NS, Hartman C, Richardson P, et al. Risk of lower and upper gastrointestinal bleeding, transfusions, and hospitalizations with complex antithrombotic therapy in elderly patients. Circulation. 2013;128:1869–77.
2. Wallentin L, Becker RC, Budaj A, et al. Ticagrelor versus clopidogrel in patients with acute coronary syndromes. N Engl J Med. 2009;361:1045–57.
3. Wiviott SD, Braunwald E, McCabe CH, et al. Prasugrel versus clopidogrel in patients with acute coronary syndromes. N Engl J Med. 2007;357:2001–15.
4. Veitch AM, Vanbiervliet G, Gershlick AH, et al. Endoscopy in patients on antiplatelet or anticoagulant therapy, including direct oral anticoagulants: British Society of Gastroenterology (BSG) and European Society of Gastrointestinal Endoscopy (ESGE) guidelines. Endoscopy. 2016;48(4):385–402.
5. Sawhney MS, Salfiti N, Nelson DB, et al. Risk factors for severe delayed postpolypectomy bleeding. Endoscopy. 2008;40:115–9.
6. Rutter MD, Nickerson C, Rees CJ, et al. Risk factors for adverse events related to polypectomy in the English Bowel Cancer Screening Programme. Endoscopy. 2014;46:90–7.
7. Choung BS, Kim SH, Ahn DS, et al. Incidence and risk factors of delayed postpolypectomy bleeding: a retrospective cohort study. J Clin Gastroenterol. 2014;48:784–9.
8. Gimeno-Garcia AZ, de Ganzo ZA, Sosa AJ, et al. Incidence and predictors of postpolypectomy bleeding in colorectal polyps larger than 10 mm. Eur J Gastroenterol Hepatol. 2012;24:520–6.
9. Kim JH, Lee HJ, Ahn JW, et al. Risk factors for delayed post-polypectomy hemorrhage: a case-control study. J Gastroenterol Hepatol. 2013;28:645–9.
10. Manocha D, Singh M, Mehta N, et al. Bleeding risk after invasive procedures in aspirin/NSAID users: polypectomy study in veterans. Am J Med. 2012;125:1222–7.
11. Repici A, Hassan C, Vitetta E, et al. Safety of cold polypectomy for <10mm polyps at colonoscopy: a prospective multicenter study. Endoscopy. 2012;44:27–31.
12. Zhang Q, An S, Chen Z, et al. Assessment of risk factors for delayed colonic post-polypectomy hemorrhage: a study of 15553 polypectomies from 2005 to 2013. PLoS One. 2014;9:e108290.
13. Burgess NG, Metz AJ, Williams SJ, et al. Risk factors for intraprocedural and clinically significant delayed bleeding after wide-field endoscopic mucosal resection of large colonic lesions. Clin Gastroenterol Hepatol. 2014;12:651–61. e1–e3
14. Kim HS, Kim TI, Kim WH, et al. Risk factors for immediate postpolypectomy bleeding of the colon: a multicenter study. Am J Gastroenterol. 2006;101:1333–41.
15. Cipolletta L, Rotondano G, Bianco MA, et al. Endoscopic resection for superficial colorectal neoplasia in Italy: a prospective multicentre study. Dig Liver Dis. 2014;46:146–51.
16. Heresbach D, Kornhauser R, Seyrig JA, et al. A national survey of endoscopic mucosal resection for superficial gastrointestinal neoplasia. Endoscopy. 2010;42:806–13.
17. Cao Y, Liao C, Tan A, et al. Meta-analysis of endoscopic submucosal dissection versus endoscopic mucosal resection for tumors of the gastrointestinal tract. Endoscopy. 2009;41:751–7.
18. Friedland S, Sedehi D, Soetikno R. Colonoscopic polypectomy in anticoagulated patients. World J Gastroenterol. 2009;15:1973–6.
19. Horiuchi A, Nakayama Y, Kajiyama M, et al. Removal of small colorectal polyps in anticoagulated patients: a prospective randomized comparison of cold snare and conventional polypectomy. Gastrointest Endosc. 2014;79:417–23.
20. Acosta RD, Abraham NS, Chandrasekhara V, ASGE Standards of Practice Committee, et al. The management of antithrombotic agents for patients undergoing GI endoscopy. Gastrointest Endosc. 2016;83(1):3–16.
21. Douketis JD, Spyropoulos AC, Kaatz S, et al. Perioperative bridging anticoagulation in patients with atrial fibrillation. N Engl J Med. 2015;373:823–33.

22. Lip GY, Nieuwlaat R, Pisters R, et al. Refining clinical risk stratification for predicting stroke and thromboembolism in atrial fibrillation using a novel risk factor-based approach: the Euro Heart Survey on atrial fibrillation. Chest. 2010;137:263–72.
23. Douketis JD, Healey JS, Brueckmann M, et al. Perioperative bridging anticoagulation during dabigatran or warfarin interruption among patients who had an elective surgery or procedure. Substudy of the RE-LY trial. Thromb Haemost. 2015;113:625–32.
24. Stangier J, Feuring M. Using the HEMOCLOT direct thrombin inhibitor assay to determine plasma concentrations of dabigatran. Blood Coagul Fibrinolysis. 2012;23:138–43.
25. Asmis LM, Alberio L, Angelillo-Scherrer A, et al. Rivaroxaban: quantification by anti-FXa assay and influence on coagulation tests: a study in 9 Swiss laboratories. Thromb Res. 2012;129:492–8.
26. Samama MM, Contant G, Spiro TE, et al. Evaluation of the anti-factor Xa chromogenic assay for the measurement of rivaroxaban plasma concentrations using calibrators and controls. Thromb Haemost. 2012;107:379–87.
27. FDA approves Praxbind, the first reversal agent for the anticoagulant Pradaxa. http://www.fda.gov/NewsEvents/Newsroom/PressAnnouncements/ucm467300.htm. Accessed 15 Oct 2015.
28. Connolly SJ, Ezekowitz MD, Yusuf S, et al. Dabigatran versus warfarin in patients with atrial fibrillation. N Engl J Med. 2009;361:1139–51.
29. Patel MR, Mahaffey KW, Garg J, et al. Rivaroxaban versus warfarin in nonvalvular atrial fibrillation. N Engl J Med. 2011;365:883–91.
30. Abraham NS, Singh S, Alexander GC, et al. Comparative risk of gastrointestinal bleeding with dabigatran, rivaroxaban, and warfarin: population based cohort study. BMJ. 2015;350:h1857.
31. Ruff CT, Giugliano RP, Braunwald E, et al. Comparison of the efficacy and safety of new oral anticoagulants with warfarin in patients with atrial fibrillation: a meta-analysis of randomised trials. Lancet. 2014;383:955–62.
32. Cangemi DJ, Krill T, Weideman R, Cipher DJ, Spechler SJ, Feagins LA. A comparison of the rate of gastrointestinal bleeding in patients taking non-vitamin K antagonist oral anticoagulants or warfarin. Am J Gastroenterol. 2017;112:734–9. https://doi.org/10.1038/ajg.2017.39.
33. Abraham NS, Noseworthy PA, Yao X, Sangaralingham LR, Shah ND. Gastrointestinal safety of direct oral anticoagulants: a large population-based study. Gastroenterology. 2016;152:1014–22. https://doi.org/10.1053/j.gastro.2016.12.018.
34. Weitz JI, Quinlan DJ, Eikelboom JW. Periprocedural management and approach to bleeding in patients taking dabigatran. Circulation. 2012;126:2428–32.
35. Dzik WS. Reversal of drug-induced anticoagulation: old solutions and new problems. Transfusion. 2012;52(Suppl 1):25S–55S.
36. Veitch AM, Baglin TP, Gershlick AH, et al. Guidelines for the management of anticoagulant and antiplatelet therapy in patients undergoing endoscopic procedures. Gut. 2008;57:1322–9.
37. Grines CL, Bonow RO, Casey DE Jr, et al. Prevention of premature discontinuation of dual antiplatelet therapy in patients with coronary artery stents: a science advisory from the American Heart Association, American College of Cardiology, Society for Cardiovascular Angiography and Interventions, American College of Surgeons, and American Dental Association, with representation from the American College of Physicians. Circulation. 2007;115:813–8.
38. Baron TH, Kamath TS, McBane ED. New anticoagulant and antiplatelet agents: A primer for the gastroenterologist. Clin Gastrenterol Hepatol. 2014;12:187–95.
39. Korte W, Cattaneo M, Chassot PG, et al. Peri-operative management of antiplatelet therapy in patients with coronary artery disease: joint position paper by members of the working group on Perioperative Haemostasis of the Society on Thrombosis and Haemostasis Research (GTH), the working group on Perioperative Coagulation of the Austrian Society for Anesthesiology, Resuscitation and Intensive Care (ÖGARI) and the Working Group Thrombosis of the European Society for Cardiology (ESC). Thromb Haemost. 2011;105:743–9.
40. Douketis JD, Spyropoulos AC, Spencer FA, et al. American College of Chest Physicians. Perioperative management of antithrombotic therapy: Antithrombotic Therapy and Prevention of Thrombosis, 9th ed: American College of Chest Physicians Evidence-Based Clinical Practice Guidelines ½erratum in: Chest 2012;141:1129. Chest. 2012;141(Suppl):e326S–50S.
41. Hall R, Mazer CD. Antiplatelet drugs: a review of their pharmacology and management in the perioperative period. Anesth Analg. 2011;112:292–318.

42. Kalantzi KI, Tsoumani ME, Goudevenos IA, et al. Pharmacodynamic properties of anti-platelet agents: current knowledge and future perspectives. Expert Rev Clin Pharmacol. 2012;5:319–36.
43. Zullo A, Hassan C, Radaelli F. Gastrointestinal endoscopy in patients on anticoagulant therapy and antiplatelet agents. Ann Gastroenterol. 2017;30:7–14.
44. Jneid H, Anderson JL, Wright RS, et al. 2012 ACCF/AHA Focused update of the guideline for the management of patients with unstable angina/non-ST-elevation myocardial infarction (updating the 2007 guideline and replacing the 2011 focused update). JACC. 2012;60:645–81.
45. Daemen J, Wenaweser P, Tsuchida K, et al. Early and late coronary stent thrombosis of sirolimus-eluting and paclitaxel-eluting stents in routine clinical practice: data from a large two-institutional cohort study. Lancet. 2007;369:667–78.
46. Becker RC, Scheiman J, Dauerman HL, et al. Management of platelet directed pharmacother-apy in patients with atherosclerotic coronary artery disease undergoing elective endoscopic gastrointestinal procedures. Am J Gastroenterol. 2009;104:2903–17.
47. Hui AJ, Wong RM, Ching JY, et al. Risk of colonoscopic polypectomy bleeding with antico-agulants and antiplatelet agents: analysis of 1657 cases. Gastrointest Endosc. 2004;59:44–8.
48. Bahin FF, Naidoo M, Williams SJ, et al. Prophylactic endoscopic coagulation to prevent bleeding after wide-field endoscopic mucosal resection of large sessile colon polyps. Clin Gastroenterol Hepatol. 2015;13:724–30. e1–e2
49. Metz AJ, Bourke MJ, Moss A, et al. Factors that predict bleeding following endoscopic muco-sal resection of large colonic lesions. Endoscopy. 2011;43:506–11.
50. Maulaz AB, Bezerra DC, Michel P, et al. Effect of discontinuing aspirin therapy on the risk of brain ischemic stroke. Arch Neurol. 2005;62:1217–20.
51. Eisenberg MJ, Richard PR, Libersan D, et al. Safety of short-term discontinuation of antiplate-let therapy in patients with drug-eluting stents. Circulation. 2009;119:1634–42.
52. Steinberg ZL, Eisen GM, Steinberg WM. Warfarin and clopidogrel interruption before and after colonoscopic polypectomy: results of a survey from a US National Audience. J Clin Gastroenterol. 2012;46:802–3.
53. Gandhi S, Narula N, Mosleh W, et al. Meta-analysis: colonoscopic post-procedural bleeding in patients on continued clopidogrel therapy. Aliment Pharmacol Ther. 2013;37:947–52.
54. Terasaki M, Tanaka S, Shigita K, et al. Risk factors for delayed bleeding after endoscopic submucosal dissection for colorectal neoplasms. Int J Color Dis. 2014;29:877–82.
55. Suzuki S, Chino A, Kishihara T, et al. Risk factors for bleeding after endoscopic submucosal dissection of colorectal neoplasms. World J Gastroenterol. 2014;20:1839–45.

Endoscopic Surveillance After Polypectomy

10

Giuseppe Galloro, Donato Alessandro Telesca,
Teresa Russo, Simona Ruggiero, and Cesare Formisano

10.1 Introduction

In Western countries, colorectal cancer (CRC) represents the second cause of cancer mortality, after lung tumors [1–3]. Its incidence is increasing in Eastern countries too, because of *westernization* of eating habits and aging of the population [4]. It seems obvious that CRC screening by colonoscopy in asymptomatic patients, being able to diagnose precancerous lesions or CRC at an early stage, may reduce either incidence or mortality [5–10]. In fact, since the mid-80s we are experiencing a sharp decline in CRC incidence in Western countries, mainly due to CRC screening programs [11]. Meanwhile, the westernization of lifestyle in the East, particularly in terms of dietary habits, has been marked since 1950 and is supposed to be directly responsible of the rising incidence of CRC [12]. Adenomatous polyps are the most common neoplastic lesions found during screening colonoscopy [13, 14], and patients with adenomatous polyps are well known to present with a significantly increased risk to develop an advanced neoplasia particularly if adenomas are larger than 10 mm or with unfavorable histology [15, 16]. Therefore, there is evidence that detection and removal of these precancerous lesions may prevent advanced CRC occurrence, reducing mortality and morbidity [17]. Moreover, patients with adenomas diagnosed at colonoscopy have an increased risk for developing metachronous adenomas and consequently cancers compared with patients without adenomas because of missed lesions or not radically removed at endoscopic examination [18–21]. This data shows the relevance of an adequate screening program for CRC and even more of a surveillance program after endoscopic polypectomy. In facts, patients who are not entered into a surveillance program present a three- or fourfold increased risk of CRC occurrence [5, 22–26]. Until the early 1990s, no surveillance guidelines

G. Galloro (✉) • D.A. Telesca • T. Russo • S. Ruggiero • C. Formisano
Department of Clinical Medicine and Surgery, Surgical Digestive Endoscopy Unit,
University of Naples Federico II – School of Medicine, Naples, Italy
e-mail: giuseppe.galloro@unina.it

© Springer International Publishing AG 2018
A. Facciorusso, N. Muscatiello (eds.), *Colon Polypectomy*,
https://doi.org/10.1007/978-3-319-59457-6_10

135

were available to address how clinicians should follow-up post-polypectomy patients. Only in 1993, the findings of a randomized trial comparing 1-year versus 3-year surveillance intervals after polypectomy (the American National Polyp Study) [27] allowed the delivery of modern guidelines in this field. Based on the American guidelines, several European countries developed their own guidelines, thus pushing the launch of broad population-based screening programs. Japan, conversely, has not yet developed specific guidelines, waiting for the conclusion of a Japanese national polyp study started in 2014.

Surveillance colonoscopies absorb about 20% of endoscopic resources in Europe (approximately the same proportion as primary screening examinations) [28, 29] and in South Korea represent the major indication to colonoscopy [4] resulting in an expensive practice for national health systems. Moreover, although colonoscopy is considered a safe procedure, it is invasive and may lead to potentially serious complications though [30]. Due to all these financial and clinical reasons, the need of an appropriate post-polypectomy surveillance program is hence mandatory.

Epidemiological and clinical studies demonstrate the possibility of a risk stratification for CRC and adenoma recurrence, identifying different subgroups of patients based on the baseline features of the resected polyps [31–37]. Many countries developed their own guidelines to reach the best balance between benefits and drawbacks of post-polypectomy surveillance in terms of lower incidence of CRC and economic impact. In general, the common attitude is to follow all the American and European studies which led to develop the respective guidelines, sharing their recommendations and slightly modifying the interval indications. One exception is represented by the Japanese endoscopic society that, although sharing the scientific bases posed by the Western studies, comes to different conclusion.

The aim of this chapter is to review the Western guidelines from the American Gastroenterological Association (AGA), American Society for Gastrointestinal Endoscopy (ASGE), and European Society for Gastrointestinal Endoscopy (ESGE) and the Eastern ones from the Japanese Society of Gastroenterological Endoscopy and Korean Society of Gastrointestinal Endoscopy (KSGE).

10.2   The Western Point of View (AGA, ASGE, and ESGE Guidelines)

The most recent edition of American and European guidelines was delivered in 2012. Both of them are very similar, since they are based on the same background principles, come to similar conclusions, and point out the importance of a quality baseline colonoscopy. Specifically, quality baseline colonoscopy is considered a procedure performed with optimal bowel preparation that allows detecting lesions of 5 mm at least, with a cecal intubation rate of 95% or more, and conducted by an expert endoscopist with an appropriate adenoma detection rate (ADR). In fact, cancer registries report up to 9% of CRCs as interval cancers in patients who underwent a colonoscopy within 6–36 months before diagnosis [38, 39]. Several studies [5,

21–25] demonstrated that interval cancers are more likely to be located in proximal compared to distal colon segments. This data seems to suggest that proximal colorectal lesions are easily missed because of incomplete examination of all colon segments, likelihood of poor quality bowel preparation in cecum and ascending colon, and higher incidence of flat and depressed non-polypoid lesions more difficult to detect in the proximal colon segments. Moreover, proximal colorectal adenomas could be biologically different comparing to distal ones, showing a shorter time of progression to malignancies.

Anyway, some studies [40–45] demonstrated that up to 17% of lesions larger than 10 mm are missed at baseline endoscopy, validating the relevance of a high-quality baseline colonoscopy.

Another important point of discussion concerns the incomplete resection of lesions detected during baseline colonoscopy. About 19–27% of interval cancers occur in the same segment of the colon as the site of a prior polypectomy, and about 17.6% of large (more than 20 mm) sessile resected polyps presented residual adenomatous tissue after polypectomy [45–47]. As a consequence, it is very important to discriminate different situations in order to stratify the potential risk of developing an interval cancer based on different baseline polyp features.

Mainly, both American [48] and European [49] current guidelines individuate two risk groups, based on the likelihood of developing advanced neoplasia after baseline colonoscopy, each including some subgroups:

1. Low-risk group
   (a) No polyps detected.
   (b) Distal polyps detected, less than 10 mm in diameter, showing hyperplastic histology.
   (c) At least two adenomas detected, less than 10 mm in diameter, showing tubular histology without dysplasia or with low-grade dysplasia.
2. High-risk group
   (a) Three to ten adenomas detected.
   (b) More than ten adenomas detected.
   (c) One or more adenomas detected, at least 10 mm in diameter, showing tubular histology.
   (d) One or more adenomas detected, of any size, showing villous histology.
   (e) One or more adenomas detected, of any size, showing high-grade dysplasia.
   (f) Serrated polyps.
   (g) Serrated polyposis syndrome.

Based on this risk stratification, it has been possible to develop different recommendations for post-polypectomy surveillance. The proper decision on the timing of surveillance takes into account the stratified risk to develop an interval cancer in a patient who underwent colorectal polypectomy, evaluated on the basis of the baseline endoscopic findings.

10.2.1 Low-Risk Group

Baseline colonoscopy: no adenoma or polyp detected—quality of evidence moderate
[48, 49]

Several prospective observational studies [7, 50, 51] demonstrated that the risk of advanced adenoma within 5 years after negative colonoscopy is slow (1.3–2.4%), and interval cancers are rare. Case control and observational studies [5, 22, 52, 53] suggested that patients with a baseline negative colonoscopy experience either reduced CRC incidence and mortality within 10 years from index colonoscopy. Recommendation is to repeat colonoscopy after 10 years and to reduce to 5 years this interval in the case of a first-degree relative with a CRC or high-risk adenoma diagnosed before 60 years.

Baseline colonoscopy: distal polyps detected, less than 10 mm in diameter, showing hyperplastic histology—quality of evidence moderate [48, 49]

Small rectal or sigmoid hyperplastic polyps are non-neoplastic lesions; hence, being at low risk of recurrence, they need only an endoscopic follow-up at 10 years.

Baseline colonoscopy: at least two adenomas detected, less than 10 mm in diameter, showing tubular histology without dysplasia or with low-grade dysplasia—quality of evidence moderate [48, 49]

Several studies [54–59] suggested that patients with one to two tubular adenomas with low-grade dysplasia <10 mm represent a low-risk group, without significant increase in risk of advanced neoplasia within 5 years. In this group, colonoscopy follow-up is indicated between 5 and 10 years according to the American guidelines and definitely at 10 years according to the European guidelines. The two guidelines slightly differ in this regard because American society [48] takes into account the risk of a poor quality examination, which is conversely strongly excluded in the European guidelines [49].

When should further surveillance after first follow-up colonoscopy be scheduled in low-risk patients? Current guidelines suggest as follows:

– At 3 years if first follow-up colonoscopy showed a high-risk condition
– At 5 years if first follow-up colonoscopy showed a low-risk condition
– At 10 years if first follow-up colonoscopy showed no adenoma

10.2.2 High-Risk Group

Baseline colonoscopy: three to ten adenomas detected—quality of evidence moderate if any polyp is ≥6 mm; quality of evidence low if any polyp is <6 mm [48, 49]

Two meta-analyses [59, 60] showed that patients with three or more adenomas at baseline colonoscopy have an increased relative risk for adenomas during surveillance, ranging from 1.7 to 4.8, mainly due to the high probability to have missed lesions at baseline exploration. This consideration suggests a more cautious approach to follow-up. Recommendation is for a 3-year interval.

Baseline colonoscopy: more than 10 adenomas detected—quality of evidence moderate-high [48, 49]

This condition is relatively rare and represents a small proportion of patients who underwent screening colonoscopy for hereditary syndromes. Since there is little evidence about this condition, follow-up is based on clinical evaluations and is suggested within 3 years.

Baseline colonoscopy: one or more adenomas detected, at least 10 mm in diameter, showing tubular histology—quality of evidence high [48, 49]

An interesting study [54] analyzed polyp size as a risk factor for development of interval advanced neoplasia. Patients with adenomas 10–19 mm in diameter at baseline colonoscopy compared with adenomas <5 mm resulted at higher risk (15.9% vs. 7.7%) due to the lower R0 resection rate. If baseline polyp was 20 mm or more, the risk rose to 19.3%. Recommendation is for follow-up at 3 years.

Baseline colonoscopy: one or more adenomas detected, of any size, showing villous histology—quality of evidence moderate [48, 49]

Compared with patients with tubular adenomas, those with villous or tubulo-villous histology have an increased risk of advanced neoplasia during follow-up (16.8% vs. 9.7%) [54]. Therefore, a 3-year follow-up is recommended. The available studies do not separately identify patients whose most advanced polyp is a tubulo-villous or villous adenoma less than 10 mm in diameter. Further studies should identify risk level based on both histology and polyp dimension.

Baseline colonoscopy: one or more adenomas detected of any size, showing high-grade dysplasia—quality of evidence moderate [48, 49]

An important study demonstrated that high-grade dysplasia is strongly associated to the risk of advanced neoplasia during surveillance (Odds ratio: 1.77; 95% CI, 1.41–2.22) [54]. Recommendation is for 3-year follow-up.

Baseline colonoscopy: serrated polyps—quality of evidence low [48, 49]

A total of 20–30% of CRC arise through a molecular pathway characterized by hypermethylation of genes known as CpG island methylator phenotype (CIMP) [26]. Precursors are considered to be serrated polyps. This kind of tumor frequently shows mutations in the B-Raf proto-oncogene serine/threonine kinase (BRAF) with up to 50% of unstableness of microsatellites. Main precursor of hypermethylated cancers is the sessile serrated polyp (or serrated adenoma). This situation indicates a more advanced lesion in the adenoma-carcinoma sequence [7]. These lesions are very difficult to detect by endoscopy. They are often small, sessile, or flat in shape, with the same color of surrounding mucosa and indistinctive edges. Mucolisis by n-acetylcysteine removes adherent mucus that, otherwise, does not allow the evaluation of glandular and vascular pattern of the lesion. Then chromoendoscopy by indigo carmine 0.4% and zoom endoscopy enable the endoscopist to find the II-O pit pattern which is highly suggestive of serrated adenomas [61, 62].

There is low-quality evidence about surveillance intervals for this kind of lesions. Based on available data, a stricter follow-up schedule should be considered for serrated adenomas larger than 10 mm in diameter, proximal to the sigmoid colon, and with dysplasia. Conversely, we have to consider serrated polyps less than 10 mm in diameter, distal to sigmoid colon and without dysplasia as low-risk adenomas.

Baseline colonoscopy: serrated polyposis syndrome—quality of evidence moderate [48, 49]

Based on the World Health Organization statement, serrated polyposis syndrome is defined by at least one of the following criteria:

1. At least five serrated adenomas proximal to sigmoid colon, with at least $2 \geq 10$ mm in diameter
2. Any serrated adenomas proximal to sigmoid colon with family history of serrated polyposis syndrome
3. More than 20 serrated adenomas of any size throughout the colon

Serrated polyposis syndrome is considered as a very high-risk condition; hence, yearly surveillance is recommended.

When should further surveillance after first follow-up colonoscopy in high-risk patients be scheduled? Current guidelines suggest as follows:

– At 3 years if first follow-up colonoscopy showed a high-risk condition
– At 5 years if first follow-up colonoscopy showed a low-risk condition
– At 5 years if first follow-up colonoscopy showed no adenoma

10.2.3 Further General Considerations [48, 49]

1. All above evaluated considerations are valid provided that high-quality baseline colonoscopy was performed. In the case of poor bowel preparation or incomplete examination, a new control is recommended within 1 year.
2. In the case of piecemeal resection of adenomas >10 mm, follow-up is recommended within 6 months before starting an appropriate surveillance program.
3. During the endoscopic surveillance program, fecal occult blood test (FOBT) is neither useful nor recommended.
4. Considerable evidence [63, 64] confirms that colonoscopy-related adverse events increase with advanced age. Therefore, surveillance and screening should be interrupted when risk outweighs benefit [60]. American guidelines suggest the age of 85 to interrupt the surveillance program [48], while European guidelines lower the threshold to 80 [49]. However, the decision to continue surveillance in old patients should be individualized, based on the assessment of benefits, risks, and comorbidities.
5. Development of new symptoms as change in bowel habits, abdominal pain, and minor rectal bleeding during the follow-up interval does not represent a cause to shorten the surveillance interval. In fact, likelihood of adenoma occurrence after a prior complete and adequate colonoscopy is uncertain but likely to be low.
6. CRC risk varies, based on patient demographic characteristics (age, race, gender), but there are no evidences that surveillance protocol should be modified once patients have performed colonoscopy or polypectomy based on these factors.

10.3 A View to the East (JSGE and KSG Guidelines)

In Eastern countries, due to westernization of habits and increasing obesity, CRC currently represents the third leading cause of cancer death in Japan and particularly the leading cause for women [65]. Eastern guidelines are mainly based on Western literature and guidelines; hence, Japanese and Korean endoscopists, gastroenterologists, and surgeons agree on the aforementioned risk stratification identifying a low- and a high-risk group. However, Eastern endoscopists further emphasize the importance of the quality of baseline colonoscopy, with particular reference to bowel preparation protocol and use of augmented endoscopy to improve the adenoma detection rate. Bowel cleansing is carried out by means of polyethylene glycol (PEG) solution administered in the morning of the day of the procedure. Moreover, standard chromoendoscopy, computed virtual chromoendoscopy (Olympus NBI, Fujinon FICE, Pentax iSCAN), and zoom magnification are regularly utilized to better detect diminutive polyps or non-polypoid lesions, according to Paris classification [65–68].

The role of colorectal post-polypectomy surveillance in Japan is not well defined and codified currently as in Western countries, and there is a lack of real and complete guidelines about it. Anyway, because of the increasing number of colorectal polyps diagnosed and endoscopically resected, there is a pressing need for clinical guidelines in this field. Therefore, the Japanese Gastroenterological Association (JGA), the Japanese Society of Gastrointestinal Cancer Screening (JSGCS), the Japan Gastroenterological Endoscopy Society (JGES), the Japan Society of Coloproctology (JSCP), and the Japanese Society for Cancer of the Colon and Rectum (JSCCR) published a common document called *Evidence-based clinical guidelines for management of colorectal polyps* that consider: (1) epidemiology; (2) screening; (3) pathophysiology, definition, and classification; (4) diagnosis; (5) treatment and management; (6) practical treatment; (7) complication and surveillance after treatment; and (8) other colorectal lesions (submucosal tumors, nonneoplastic polyps, polyposis, hereditary tumors, ulcerative colitis-associated tumor/cancer) [69]. It should be noted that surveillance is just a chapter of the entire document.

However, although these guidelines speculatively follow the Western recommendations, indeed they come to different conclusions. First, remarkable difference is about the management of detected lesions. While the trend in the West is to remove every kind of detected lesion regardless of size (obviously excepting for hyperplastic lesions), Japanese recommendation is not to resect diminutive (less than 5 mm in diameter) adenomatous lesions, excluding flat and depressed non-polypoid lesions and then establish an annual follow-up for 3 years [15, 70–73].

Other key difference is that, unlike Western recommendations, the indication is for a 3-year follow-up schedule after polypectomy of any kind of lesion [69, 74].

Korean guidelines [75], given the lack of definitive assumptions based on the current literature, endorse the Western approach with the stratification into two risk groups: 5-year follow-up for patients with no high-risk feature at baseline colonoscopy and 3-year follow-up for patients with one or more high-risk features at baseline colonoscopy.

References

1. Ferlay J, Autier P, Boniol M, et al. Estimates of the cancer incidence and mortality in Europe in 2006. Ann Oncol. 2007;18:581–92. Epub 2007 Feb 7
2. Edwards BK, Ward E, Kohler BA, et al. Annual report to the nation on the status of cancer, 1975–2006, featuring colorectal cancer trends and impact of interventions (risk factors, screening, and treatment) to reduce future rates. Cancer. 2010;116:544–73.
3. Joseph DA, King JB, Miller JW, et al. Prevalence of colorectal cancer screening among adults – behavioral risk factor surveillance system, United States, 2010. Morb Mortal Wkly Rep. 2012;61:51–6.
4. Tae OK. Optimal colonoscopy surveillance interval after polypectomy. Clin Endosc. 2016;49:359–63.
5. Baxter NN, Goldwasser MA, Paszat LF, et al. Association of colonoscopy and death from colorectal cancer. Ann Intern Med. 2009;150:1–8.
6. Hewitson P, Glasziou P, Irwig L, et al. Screening for colorectal cancer using the faecal occult blood test, hemoccult. Cochrane Database Syst Rev. 2007;(1):CD001216.
7. Atkin WS, Edwards R, Kralj-Hans I, et al. Once-only flexible sigmoidoscopy screening in prevention of colorectal cancer: a multicentre randomised controlled trial. Lancet. 2010;375:1624–33.
8. von Karsa L, Patnick J, Segnan N. European guidelines for quality assurance in colorectal cancer screening and diagnosis. First Edition – executive summary. Endoscopy. 2012;44(Suppl 3):SE1–8.
9. Atkin W, Kralj-Hans I, Wardle J, et al. Colorectal cancer screening. Randomised trials of flexible sigmoidoscopy. BMJ. 2010;341:c4618.
10. Kahi CJ, Imperiale TF, Juliar BE, et al. Effect of screening colonoscopy on colorectal cancer incidence and mortality. Clin Gastroenterol Hepatol. 2009;7:770–5.
11. Nelson RL, Persky V, Turyk M. Determination of factors responsible for the declining incidence of colorectal cancers. Dis Colon Rectum. 1999;42:741–52.
12. Kuriki K, Tajima K. The increasing incidence of colorectal cancer and the preventive strategy in Japan. Asian Pac J Cancer Prev. 2006;7:495–501.
13. Liebermann DA, Weiss DG, Bond JH, Ahnen DJ, et al. Use of colonoscopy to screen asymptomatic adults for colorectal cancer. Veterans affairs cooperative study group 380. N Engl J Med. 2000;343:162–1688.
14. Schoenfeld P, Cash B, Flood A, et al. Colonoscopic screening of average risk women for colorectal neoplasia. N Engl J Med. 2005;352:2061–8.
15. Yamaji Y, Mitsushima T, Ikuma H, et al. Incidence and recurrence rates of colorectal adenomas estimated by annually repeated colonoscopies on asymptomatic Japanese. Gut. 2004;53:568–72.
16. Cottet V, Jooste V, Fournel I, et al. Long-term risk of colorectal cancer after adenoma removal: a population-based cohort study. Gut. 2012;61:1180–6.
17. Zauber AG, Winawer SJ, O'Brien MJ, et al. Colonoscopic polypectomy and long-term prevention of colorectal-cancer deaths. N Engl J Med. 2012;366:687–96.
18. Robertson DJ, Greenberg ER, Beach M, et al. Colorectal cancer in patients under close colonoscopic surveillance. Gastroenterology. 2005;129:34–41.
19. Loeve F, van Ballegooijen M, Boer R, et al. Colorectal cancer risk in adenoma patients: a nation-wide study. Int J Cancer. 2004;111:147–51.
20. Rex DK, Cutler CS, Lemmel GT, et al. Colonoscopic miss rates of adenomas determined by back-to-back colonoscopies. Gastroenterology. 1997;112:24–8.
21. Anti M, Armuzzi A, Morini S, et al. Severe imbalance of cell proliferation and apoptosis in the left colon and in the rectosigmoid tract in subjects with a history of large adenomas. Gut. 2001;48:238–46.
22. Singh H, Turner D, Xue L, et al. Risk of developing colorectal cancer following a negative colonoscopy examination. JAMA. 2006;295:2366–73.

23. Bressler B, Paszat LF, Chen Z, et al. Rates of new or missed colorectal cancers after colonos-copy and their risk factors: a population-based analysis. Gastroenterology. 2007;132:96–102.
24. Lakoff J, Paszat LF, Saskin R, et al. Risk of developing proximal versus distal colorectal cancer after a negative colonoscopy: a population-based study. Clin Gastroenterol Hepatol. 2008;6:1117–21.
25. Brenner H, Chang-Claude J, Seiler CM, et al. Protection from colorectal cancer after colonos-copy. Ann Intern Med. 2011;154:22–30.
26. Leggett B, Whitehall V. Role of the serrated pathway in colorectal cancer pathogenesis. Gastroenterology. 2010;138:2088–100.
27. Winawer SJ, Zauber AG, O'Brien MJ, et al. Randomized comparison of surveillance inter-vals after colonoscopic removal of newly diagnosed adenomatous polyps. The National Polyp Study Workgroup. N Engl J Med. 1993;328:901–6.
28. Radaelli F, Paggi S, Bortoli A, et al. Overutilization of post-polypectomy surveillance colonos-copy in clinical practice: a prospective, multicentre study. Dig Liver Dis. 2012;44:748–53.
29. Lieberman DA, Holub J, Eisen G, et al. Utilization of colonoscopy in the United States: results from a national consortium. Gastrointest Endosc. 2005;62:875–83.
30. Levy I, Gralner IM, et al. Complications of diagnostic colonoscopy, upper endoscopy and enteroscopy. Best Pract Res Clin Gastroenterol. 2016;30(5):705–18.
31. Atkin WS, Morson BC, Cuzick J. Long-term risk of colorectal cancer after excision of recto-sigmoid adenomas. N Engl J Med. 1992;326:658–62.
32. Brenner H, Chang-Claude J, Rickert A, et al. Risk of colorectal cancer after detection and removal of adenomas at colonoscopy: population-based case-control study. J Clin Oncol. 2012;30:2969–76.
33. Regula J, Rupinski M, Kraszewska E, et al. Colonoscopy in colorectal-cancer screening for detection of advanced neoplasia. N Engl J Med. 2006;355:1863–72.
34. Hassan C, Pickhardt PJ, Kim DH, et al. Systematic review: distribution of advanced neoplasia according to polyp size at screening colonoscopy. Aliment Pharmacol Ther. 2010;31:210–7.
35. Gupta N, Bansal A, Rao D, et al. Prevalence of advanced histological features in diminutive and small colon polyps. Gastrointest Endosc. 2012;75:1022–30.
36. Kahi CJ, Hewett DG, Norton DL, et al. Prevalence and variable detection of proximal colon serrated polyps during screening colonoscopy. Clin Gastroenterol Hepatol. 2011;9:42–6.
37. Rex DK, Overhiser AJ, Chen SC, et al. Estimation of impact of American College of Radiology recommendations on CT colonography reporting for resection of high-risk adenoma findings. Am J Gastroenterol. 2009;104:149–53.
38. Baxter NN, Sutradhar R, Forbes SS, et al. Analysis of administrative data finds endosco-pist quality measures associate with post-colonoscopy colorectal cancer. Gastroenterology. 2011;140:65–72.
39. Singh H, Nugent Z, Demers AA, et al. Rate and predictors of early/missed colorectal cancers after colonoscopy in Manitoba: a population-based study. Am J Gastroenterol. 2010;105:2588–96.
40. Rockey DC, Paulson E, Niedzwiecki D, et al. Analysis of air contrast barium enema, com-puted tomographic colonography and colonoscopy: prospective comparison. Lancet. 2005;365:305–11.
41. Graser A, Stieber P, Nagel D, et al. Comparison of CT colonography, colonoscopy, sigmoid-oscopy and faecal occult blood tests for the detection of advanced adenoma in an average risk population. Gut. 2009;58:241–8.
42. Cotton PB, Durkalski VL, Pineau BC, et al. Computed tomographic colonography (virtual colonoscopy): a multicenter comparison with standard colonoscopy for detection of colorectal neoplasia. JAMA. 2004;291:1713–9.
43. Benson M, Dureja P, Gopal D, Reichelderfer M, Pfau PR. A comparison of optical colonos-copy and CT colonography screening strategies in the detection and recovery of subcentimeter adenomas. Am J Gastroenterol. 2010;105:2578–85.
44. Pohl H, Robertson DJ. Colorectal cancers detected after colonoscopy frequently result from missed lesions. Clin Gastroenterol Hepatol. 2010;8:858–64.

45. Robertson DJ, Lieberman DA, Winawer SJ, et al. Interval cancer after total colonoscopy: results from a pooled analysis of eight studies. Gastroenterology. 2008;134:A111–2.
46. Pabby A, Schoen RE, Weissfeld JL, et al. Analysis of colorectal cancer occurrence during surveillance colonoscopy in the dietary polyp prevention trial. Gastrointest Endosc. 2005;61:385–91.
47. Khashab M, Eid E, Rusche M, et al. Incidence and predictors of "late" recurrences after endoscopic piecemeal resection of large sessile adenomas. Gastrointest Endosc. 2009;70:344–9.
48. Lieberman DA, Rex DK, Winawer SJ, et al. Guidelines for colonoscopy surveillance after screening and polypectomy: a consensus update by the US multi-society task force on colorectal cancer. Gastroenterology. 2012;143:844–52.
49. Hassan C, et al. Post-polypectomy colonoscopy surveillance: European society of gastrointestinal endoscopy (ESGE) guideline. Endoscopy. 2013;45:842–53.
50. Imperiale TF, Glowinski EA, Lin-Cooper C, et al. Five-year risk of colorectal neoplasia after negative screening colonoscopy. N Engl J Med. 2008;359(12):1218–24.
51. Chung SJ, Kim YS, Yang SY, et al. Five-year risk for advanced colorectal neoplasia after initial colonoscopy according to the baseline risk stratification: a prospective study in 2452 asymptomatic Koreans. Gut. 2011;60:1537–43.
52. Brenner H, Haug U, Arndt V, et al. Low risk of colorectal cancer and advanced adenomas more than 10 years after negative colonoscopy. Gastroenterology. 2010;138:870–6.
53. Brenner H, Change-Claude J, Seiler CM, et al. Long-term risk of colorectal cancer after negative colonoscopy. J Clin Oncol. 2011;29:3761–7.
54. Martinez ME, Baron JA, Lieberman DA, et al. A pooled analysis of advanced colorectal neoplasia diagnoses following colonoscopic polypectomy. Gastroenterology. 2009;136:832–41.
55. Arber N, Eagle CJ, Spicak J, et al. Celecoxib for the prevention of colorectal adenomatous polyps. N Engl J Med. 2006;355:885–95.
56. Miller H, Mukherjee R, Tian J, et al. Colonoscopy surveillance after polypectomy may be extended beyond five years. J Clin Gastroenterol. 2010;44:e162–6.
57. Laiyemo AO, Murphy W, Albert PS, et al. Post-polypectomy colonoscopy surveillance guidelines: predictive accuracy for advanced adenoma at 4 years. Ann Intern Med. 2008;148:419–26.
58. Miller J, Mehta N, Feldman M, et al. Findings on serial surveillance colonoscopy in patients with low-risk polyps on initial colonoscopy. J Clin Gastroenterol. 2010;44:e46–50.
59. Saini SD, Kim HM, Schoenfeld P. Incidence of advanced adenomas at surveillance colonoscopy in patients with a personal history of colon adenomas: a meta-analysis and systematic review. Gastrointest Endosc. 2006;64:614–26.
60. Rex DK, Kahi CJ, Levin B, Smith RA, et al. Guidelines for colonoscopy surveillance after cancer resection: a consensus update by the American Cancer Society and the US Multi-Society Task Force on Colorectal Cancer. Gastroenterology. 2006;130:1865–71.
61. Kashida H, Ikehara N, Hamatani S, Kudo SE, Kudo M. Endoscopic characteristics of colorectal serrated lesions. Hepato-Gastroenterology. 2011;58:1163–7.
62. Burke CA, Snover DC. Editorial: sessile serrated adenomas and their pit patterns: we must first see the forest through the trees. Am J Gastroenterol. 2012;107(3):470–2.
63. Warren JL, Klabunde CN, Mariotto AB, et al. Adverse events after outpatient colonoscopy in the Medicare population. Ann Intern Med. 2009;150:849–57.
64. Ko CW, Riffle S, Michaels L, et al. Serious complications within 30 days of screening and surveillance colonoscopy: a multicenter study. Clin Gastroenterol Hepatol. 2010;8:166–73.
65. Kasugai K, Ogasawara N, Sasaki M. Colonoscopy surveillance after polypectomy. Clin J Gastroenterol. 2011;4:355–63.
66. Fujii T, Rembacken BJ, Dixon MF, et al. Flat adenomas in the United Kingdom: are treatable cancers being missed? Endoscopy. 1998;30:437–43.
67. Chiu HM, Lin JT, Wang HP, et al. The impact of colon preparation timing on colonoscopic detection of colorectal neoplasms: a prospective endoscopist-blinded randomized trial. Am J Gastroenterol. 2006;101:2719–25.

68. Parra-Blanco A, Nicolas-Perez D, Gimeno-Garcia A, et al. The timing of bowel preparation before colonoscopy determines the quality of cleansing, and is a significant factor contributing to detection of flat lesions: a randomized study. World J Gastroenterol. 2006;12:6161–6.
69. Tanaka S, Saitoh Y, Matsuda T, et al. Evidence-based clinical practice guidelines for management of colorectal polyps. J Gastroenterol. 2015;50:252–60.
70. Suzuki Y, Matsuike T, Nozawa H, et al. Treatment strategy for colorectal polyps and surveillance method by total colonoscopy. Ther Res. 1997;18:S362–5.
71. Fukutomi Y, Moriwaki H, Nagase S, et al. Metachronous colon tumors: risk factors and rationale for the surveillance colonoscopy after initial polypectomy. J Cancer Res Clin Oncol. 2002;128:569–74.
72. Asano M, Matsuda Y, Kawai M, et al. Long-term outcome and surveillance after endoscopic removal for colorectal adenoma: from the viewpoint of the cases with multiple colorectal polyps. Dig Med. 2006;43:299–306.
73. Kawamura T, Ueda M, Cho E. Surveillance after colonoscopic removal of adenomatous polyps. Dig Med. 2006;43:307–10.
74. Matsuda T, Fujii T, Sano Y, et al. Five-year incidence of advanced neoplasia after initial colonoscopy in Japan: a multicenter retrospective cohort study. Jpn J Clin Oncol. 2009;39:435–42.
75. Hong SN, Yanh DH, Kim YH, et al. Korean guidelines for post-polypectomy colonoscopic surveillance. Korean J Gastroenterol. 2012;59(2):99–117.

Conclusive Remarks and New Perspectives

11

Antonio Facciorusso and Nicola Muscatiello

11.1 Introduction

Colorectal polypectomy is a well-recognized method for the prevention of colorectal cancer (CRC) through the early interruption of the adenoma-carcinoma sequence [1].

However, despite proven effectiveness, polyp resection techniques are limited by lack of evidence and are mainly based on expert opinion and uncontrolled observational studies [2].

Proper removal of polyp needs not only skillness by experienced endoscopists but also a deep knowledge of the characteristics of endoscopic equipment, according to morphology and size of the colorectal polyp, in order to avoid complications and to reduce the occurrence of incomplete polypectomy, which is one of the major causes of interval colon cancer [3, 4].

All the main CRC screening programs call for a quality colonoscopy, characterized by the detection and resection of all polypoid lesions, with subsequent submission of all resected polyps to pathologic examination [5].

As a consequence of screening programs, since the mid-1980s we are experiencing a sharp decline in CRC incidence [6].

Moreover, patients with adenomas diagnosed at colonoscopy have an increased risk for developing metachronous adenomas and consequently cancers compared with patients without adenomas; hence adequate surveillance programs after endoscopic polypectomy are mandatory [7, 8].

Aim of this book is to provide the reader with a comprehensive and up-to-date overview of this important topic.

A. Facciorusso (✉) • N. Muscatiello
Gastroenterology Unit, Department of Medical Sciences, University of Foggia,
AOU Ospedali Riuniti, Viale Pinto, 1, 71100 Foggia, Italy
e-mail: antonio.facciorusso@virgilio.it

© Springer International Publishing AG 2018
A. Facciorusso, N. Muscatiello (eds.), *Colon Polypectomy*,
https://doi.org/10.1007/978-3-319-59457-6_11

11.2   Classification of Colon Mucosal Lesions and Risk of Neoplastic Progression

The morphology of colonic lesions depends on the direction of proliferation growth.

Following this, two main macroscopic types may be recognized: superficial lesions (type 0) and advanced cancers (type 1–5) [9].

According to the Paris classification, lesions with superficial appearance (category 0) are distinguished in polypoid type (elevated more than 2.5 mm above the mucosal layer: pedunculated (0-1p), sessile (0-1s), or mixed (0-1sp)), non-polypoid (slightly elevated less than 2.5 mm (0-IIa), flat (0-IIb), or slightly depressed (0-IIc)), and mixed types [9].

Large polypoid and non-polypoid lesions (particularly if flat or depressed) are at increased risk of submucosal invasion (SMI) [9, 10].

Proper characterization of mucosal lesions requires the use of specific tools, among them chromoendoscopy or narrowband imaging (NBI) to better define particular features such as pit and vascular pattern [11–13].

Final pathological examination of the resected lesion is fundamental to correctly assess the risk of progression and recurrence, thus defining the appropriate surveillance schedule.

11.3   Methods to Improve the Adenoma Detection Rate

Studies have shown that up to 25% of adenomas are missed during colonoscopy, resulting in high interval cancer incidence [14]. In light of these observations, a high-quality examination that will ensure the detection and removal of all precancerous lesions is warranted, and so several quality-assessment indicators have been developed, such as the worldwide accepted adenoma detection rate (ADR) [15]. ADR is defined as the proportion of average-risk patients undergoing first-time screening colonoscopy in which at least one adenoma is found [15]. It has been demonstrated that an ADR that exceeds 25% is significantly associated with a reduction in interval CRC [16]. Therefore, current American Society of Gastrointestinal Endoscopy (ASGE) guidelines propose that in patients undergoing screening colonoscopy, an ADR of ≥30% in men and of ≥20% in women should be achieved [17].

Adequate bowel preparation [18] and meticulous inspection of the mucosa during scope withdrawal [19] are of paramount importance for efficient colon examination. Moreover, techniques like a second examination of the right colon either with direct or with retroflexed view [20] and water-assisted colonoscopy [21] promise better quality of the examination. Beyond these procedural issues, new endoscopic modalities including wide-angle view endoscopes and add-on devices have been developed in an effort to improve colonoscopy diagnostic yield by either expanding the field of scope view up to 330° or by providing retrograde view of the lumen or by flattening the haustral folds during withdrawal [22, 23].

In conclusion, adequate bowel preparation, sufficient withdrawal time exceeding 6 min, and second visualization of the right colon are among others easy-to-follow procedural factors that have demonstrated ADR improvement. During the last years, several endoscopic technologies have been developed to optimize visualization of the colonic mucosa. Although most of them have demonstrated impressive results regarding polyp detection, their impact in clinical practice is still questionable since all these modalities have not proved a significant impact on CRC prevention yet.

11.4 Colonoscopic Polypectomy: Current Techniques and Controversies

Successful polypectomy has to be effective in complete resection, efficient in retrieving all resected lesions, and safe in minimizing the risk of complication such as perforation or bleeding. Furthermore the resection must provide an accurate histological diagnosis.

There are several techniques to remove polyps, and the choice depends on the morphology, size, location of polyps, and the experience of the endoscopist [24].

The endoscopic techniques for resection of smaller polyps are cold forceps biopsy (CFB), hot forceps biopsy (HFB), cold or hot snare excision, and argon plasma coagulation (APC). Advanced techniques for larger lesions are endoscopic mucosal resection (EMR) and endoscopic submucosal dissection (ESD).

The optimal method to polypectomy is removing polyps in one piece (*en bloc* resection), but if the size of polyp is larger than 2 cm, resection in multiple pieces ("piecemeal resection") is the only option.

Resection techniques to treat difficult colorectal lesions include the inject-and-cut EMR, EMR with specialized cap (EMR-C), EMR with band ligation (EMR-L), underwater EMR, ESD, and specialized polypectomy techniques [25].

ESD has emerged as the approach with the greatest potentially curative yield with the major advantage being the ability to achieve *en bloc* excision for early-stage neoplasms and allowing an accurate estimation of the risk of lymph node metastasis as well as of the clearance of resection margins. Nowadays, colorectal ESD has been implemented with standard indications and is widely diffused in East Asia and Japan where *en bloc* resection is the primary target [26]. However, its application is still debated in Europe and the United States in favor of EMR because of the greater technical difficulty, longer operating times, and increased risk of perforation. However, endoscopists should be aware of the possibility of using hybrid techniques during the learning of colorectal ESD to reduce the technical challenge of completing the procedure. By the way, ESD is safe and effective when performed by experienced endoscopists, and it is reasonable to assume that its use for colorectal neoplasms will spread widely in the future given the continuous development of strategies and technology refinements.

EMR and ESD are usually performed through the injection of a fluid agent into the submucosal space to expand it, rendering polypectomy easier and safer.

Several injection solutions have been tested and are currently used to create a submucosal cushion delimiting the lesion from the muscularis propria, so allowing the complete resection of the lesion and preventing perforation and thermal injury to the gastrointestinal (GI) wall. Among them, normal saline (NS) solution is most commonly used in clinical practice because of its low cost and ease of use [26]. However, NS often requires repeated injections because of its rapid absorption into the surrounding tissue, thus increasing the risk of piecemeal resection and theoretically hampering the overall efficacy of the procedure [27].

This aspect pushed the endoscopy community to test various submucosal injection solutions such as hyaluronic acid (HA) [28], glycerol [29], dextrose water (DW) [30], fibrinogen mixture (FM) [31], polidocanol [32], and hydroxypropyl methylcellulose (HPMC) [33] in order to fulfill the pressing need of the ideal agent for EMR and ESD.

Such substances have been tested due to their ability to create a longer-lasting submucosal cushion as a result of their viscous properties. In doing so, they should be potentially able to allow lengthier procedures and increase the rate of *en bloc* resection, even for large lesions.

However, despite the promising results of the preliminary reports, their efficacy in preventing the main complication after polypectomy, namely, post-polypectomy bleeding (PPB), is still a matter of debate.

An ideal submucosal injection solution should be inexpensive, readily available, nontoxic, easy to prepare and inject, and should provide a long-lasting submucosal cushion [26]. It should also provide a sufficiently high submucosal elevation to facilitate *en bloc* resection (to reduce the local recurrence rate) and reduce the risk of perforation [26]. Unfortunately, none of the aforementioned substances seem to fulfill all of these features.

11.5   Complications of Colon Polypectomy

Colonic perforation during colonoscopy may occur as a direct result of therapeutic procedures like polypectomy. Early symptoms of perforation include persistent abdominal pain and abdominal distention. Later, patients may develop peritonitis. Surgical consultation should be obtained in all cases of perforation. Although perforation often requires surgical repair, nonsurgical management may be appropriate in selected individuals [34].

Hemorrhage is the most frequent complication of colon polypectomy, and it may occur immediately or can be delayed for several weeks after the procedure [35].

Polyp size has been reported as a risk factor for post-polypectomy bleeding (PPB) in several studies, but additional risk factors may include the number of polyps removed, recent antithrombotic therapy, and polyp histology [36].

Colon polypectomy is considered a procedure at high risk of bleeding; hence antithrombotic agents should be interrupted before the procedure, and the timing for suspension has been recently defined [37]. Of particular interest is the management of novel direct oral anticoagulant, whose timing of interruption should be defined based on renal function [37].

Post-polypectomy electrocoagulation syndrome is the result of electrocoagulation injury to the bowel wall that induces a transmural burn and localized peritonitis without evidence of perforation on radiographic studies. Typically, patients with post-polypectomy electrocoagulation syndrome present 1–5 days after colonoscopy with fever, localized abdominal pain, localized peritoneal signs, and leukocytosis [38]. It does not require surgical treatment, but it is usually managed with intravenous hydration, broad-spectrum parenteral antibiotics, and bowel rest until recovery [39].

11.6 Endoscopic Surveillance After Colon Polypectomy

Current surveillance guidelines recommend a 3-year surveillance interval for advanced colorectal adenomas (ACA) (defined by at least one of the following: ≥ 1 cm in diameter, villous component, and high-grade dysplasia (HGD), namely, those features determining a higher risk of progression to carcinoma), whereas a more delayed surveillance should be scheduled in the case of tubular adenomas <1 cm and with low-grade dysplasia (LGD) [40, 41]. These recommendations assume that the baseline colonoscopy was complete and adequate and that all visible polyps were completely removed.

However, even within each subgroup, recurrence rates vary considerably according to several baseline factors [42, 43].

Our group has recently developed a model built through a statistical method called "recursive partitioning analysis," aimed at defining three different classes of risk for ACA recurrence after polypectomy [44]. We defined as low-risk class (recurrence rate 4.2%) patients with a single ACA ≤15 mm and with LGD; medium-risk class (recurrence rate 21.3%) patients with single ACA ≤15 mm with HGD, single ACA without HGD >15 mm, or multiple ACAs without HGD ≤15 mm; and high-risk class (recurrence rate 57.9%) those patients with HGD >15 mm [44].

Based on these findings, we have recently further refined the model by developing and validating an objective numeric score derived from the aforementioned variables (namely, grade of dysplasia, number of ACA, and size) [45].

11.7 New Perspectives

Pressing evidence shows that diminutive colonic polyps ($\leq$ 5 mm) present a very low risk of cancer (0–0.6%) that justifies a "resect and discard" strategy [46], whereas for hyperplastic polyps located in the rectosigmoid, a "diagnose and leave behind" strategy is appropriate because these harbor an even lower risk of cancer [47]. In these situations, the technology used is of paramount importance since a number of novel tools are currently available such as narrowband imaging (NBI), flexible spectral imaging color enhancement (FICE), and i-SCAN digital contrast (I-SCAN) [48].

The important caveats with regard to real-time optical diagnosis concern the endoscopist's expertise in optical biopsy and degree of confidence.

Circumferential incision of lesions using ESD techniques (c- EMR, CSI-EMR, or EMR-precut) seems to allow extension of the size limits while mitigating perforation risk [49, 50]. The use of special devices such as dual-loop snares may also increase the rate of *en bloc* resection for lesions ≥20 mm to 64% [51], while underwater EMR has demonstrated *en bloc* resection rates of 55% for colorectal lesions of 20–40 mm [52].

In conclusions, like many other fields of medicine, colon polypectomy is an evolving topic. The endoscopist should be aware of the main changes in this field, particularly with regard to prevention of complications and macroscopic characterization of the lesion.

References

1. Winawer SJ, Zauber AG, Ho MN, O'Brien MJ, Gottlieb LS, Sternberg SS, Waye JD, Schapiro M, Bond JH, Panish JF. Prevention of colorectal cancer by colonoscopic polypectomy. The National Polyp Study Workgroup. N Engl J Med. 1993;329:1977–81.
2. Rex DK. Have we defined best colonoscopic polypectomy practice in the United States? Clin Gastroenterol Hepatol. 2007;5:674–7.
3. Pabby A, Schoen RE, Weissfeld JL, Burt R, Kikendall JW, Lance P, Shike M, Lanza E, Schatzkin A. Analysis of colorectal cancer occurrence during surveillance colonoscopy in the dietary polyp prevention trial. Gastrointest Endosc. 2005;61(3):385–91.
4. Farrar WD, Sawhney MS, Nelson DB, Lederle FA, Bond JH. Colorectal cancers found after a complete colonoscopy. Clin Gastroenterol Hepatol. 2006;4(10):1259–64.
5. Rembacken B, Hassan C, Riemann JF, Chilton A, Rutter M, Dumonceau JM, Omar M, Ponchon T. Quality in screening colonoscopy: position statement of the European Society of Gastrointestinal Endoscopy (ESGE). Endoscopy. 2012;44(10):957–68.
6. Nelson RL, Persky V, Turyk M. Determination of factors responsible for the declining incidence of colorectal cancers. Dis Colon Rectum. 1999;42:741–52.
7. Zauber AG, Winawer SJ, O'Brien MJ, Lansdorp-Vogelaar I, van Ballegooijen M, Hankey BF, Shi W, Bond JH, Schapiro M, Panish JF, Stewart ET, Waye JD. Colonoscopic polypectomy and long-term prevention of colorectal-cancer deaths. N Engl J Med. 2012;366:687–96.
8. Robertson DJ, Greenberg ER, Beach M, Sandler RS, Ahnen D, Haile RW, Burke CA, Snover DC, Bresalier RS, McKeown-Eyssen G, Mandel JS, Bond JH, Van Stolk RU, Summers RW, Rothstein R, Church TR, Cole BF, Byers T, Mott L, Baron JA. Colorectal cancer in patients under close colonoscopic surveillance. Gastroenterology. 2005;129:34–41.
9. Endoscopic Classification Review Group. Update on the paris classification of superficial neoplastic lesions in the digestive tract. Endoscopy. 2005;37(6):570–8.
10. Facciorusso A, Antonino M, Di Maso M, Barone M, Muscatiello N. Non-polypoid colorectal neoplasms: classification, therapy and follow-up. World J Gastroenterol. 2015;21(17):5149–57.
11. Ng SC, Lau JY. Narrow-band imaging in the colon: limitations and potentials. J Gastroenterol Hepatol. 2011;26(11):1589–96.
12. Kudo S, Hirota S, Nakajima T, Hosobe S, Kusaka H, Kobayashi T, Himori M, Yagyuu A. Colorectal tumours and pit pattern. J Clin Pathol. 1994;47(10):880–5.

13. Katagiri A, Fu KI, Sano Y, Ikematsu H, Horimatsu T, Kaneko K, Muto M, Yoshida S. Narrow band imaging with magnifying colonoscopy as diagnostic tool for predicting histology of early colorectal neoplasia. Aliment Pharmacol Ther. 2008;27(12):1269–74.
14. Heresbach D, Barrioz T, Lapalus MG, Coumaros D, Bauret P, Potier P, Sautereau D, Boustiere C, Grimaud JC, Barthelemy C, See J, Serraj I, D'Halluin PN, Branger B, Ponchon T. Miss rate for colorectal neoplastic polyps: a prospective multicenter study of back-to-back video colonoscopies. Endoscopy. 2008;40(4):284–90.
15. Triantafyllou K, Sioulas AD, Kalli T, Misailidis N, Polymeros D, Papanikolaou IS, Karamanolis G, Ladas SD. Optimized sedation improves colonoscopy quality long-term. Gastroenterol Res Pract. 2015:195093.
16. Kaminski MF, Regula J, Kraszewska E, Polkowski M, Wojciechowska U, Didkowska J, Zwierko M, Rupinski M, Nowacki MP, Butruk E. Quality indicators for colonoscopy and the risk of interval cancer. N Engl J Med. 2010;362(19):1795–803.
17. Rex DK, Schoenfeld PS, Cohen J, Pike IM, Adler DG, Fennerty MB, Lieb JG 2nd, Park WG, Rizk MK, Sawhney MS, Shaheen NJ, Wani S, Weinberg DS. Quality indicators for colonoscopy. Gastrointest Endosc. 2015;81(1):31–53.
18. Johnson DA, Barkun AN, Cohen LB, Dominitz JA, Kaltenbach T, Martel M, Robertson DJ, Boland CR, Giardello FM, Lieberman DA, Levin TR, Rex DK. Cancer USM-STFoC optimizing adequacy of bowel cleansing for colonoscopy: recommendations from the US multisociety task force on colorectal cancer. Gastroenterology. 2014;147(4):903–24.
19. Barclay RL, Vicari JJ, Doughty AS, Johanson JF, Greenlaw RL. Colonoscopic withdrawal times and adenoma detection during screening colonoscopy. N Engl J Med. 2006;355(24):2533–41.
20. Hewett DG, Rex DK. Miss rate of right-sided colon examination during colonoscopy defined by retroflexion: an observational study. Gastrointest Endosc. 2011;74(2):246–52.
21. Leung FW, Amato A, Ell C, Friedland S, Harker JO, Hsieh YH, Leung JW, Mann SK, Paggi S, Pohl J, Radaelli F, Ramirez FC, Siao-Salera R, Terruzzi V. Water-aided colonoscopy: a systematic review. Gastrointest Endosc. 2012;76(3):657–66.
22. Gralnek IM, Siersema PD, Halpern Z, Segol O, Melhem A, Suissa A, Santo E, Sloyer A, Fenster J, Moons LM, Dik VK, D'Agostino RB Jr, Rex DK. Standard forward-viewing colonoscopy versus full-spectrum endoscopy: an international, multicentre, randomised, tandem colonoscopy trial. Lancet Oncol. 2014;15(3):353–60.
23. Rastogi A, Bansal A, Rao DS, Gupta N, Wani SB, Shipe T, Gaddam S, Singh V, Sharma P. Higher adenoma detection rates with cap-assisted colonoscopy: a randomised controlled trial. Gut. 2012;61(3):402–8.
24. Bourke M. Current status of colonic endoscopic mucosal resection in the west and the interface with endoscopic submucosal dissection. Dig Endosc. 2009;21(suppl 1):S22–7.
25. Burgess NG, Bourke MJ. Endoscopic resection of colorectal lesions: the narrowing divide between east and west. Dig Endosc. 2016;28(3):296–305.
26. Sanchez-Yague A, Kaltenbach T, Raju G, Soetikno R. Advanced endoscopic resection of colorectal lesions. Gastroenterol Clin N Am. 2013;42(3):459–77.
27. Kedia P, Waye JD. Routine and advanced polypectomy techniques. Curr Gastroenterol Rep. 2011;13:506–11.
28. Kishihara T, Chino A, Uragami N, Yoshizawa N, Imai M, Ogawa T, Igarashi M. Usefulness of sodium hyaluronate solution in colorectal endoscopic mucosal resection. Dig Endosc. 2012;24(5):348–52.
29. Uraoka T, Fujii T, Saito Y, Sumiyoshi T, Emura F, Bhandari P, Matsuda T, Fu KI, Saito D. Effectiveness of glycerol as a submucosal injection for EMR. Gastrointest Endosc. 2005;61:736–40.
30. Katsinelos P, Kountouras J, Paroutoglou G, Chatzimavroudis G, Zavos C, Pilpilidis I, Gelas G, Paikos D, Karakousis K. A comparative study of 50% dextrose and normal saline solution on their ability to create submucosal fluid cushions for endoscopic resection of sessile rectosigmoid polyps. Gastrointest Endosc. 2008;68:692–8.

31. Lee SH, Park JH, Park do H, Chung IK, Kim HS, Park SH, Kim SJ, Cho HD. Clinical efficacy of EMR with submucosal injection of a fibrinogen mixture: a prospective randomized trial. Gastrointest Endosc. 2006;64:691–6.

32. Facciorusso A, Di Maso M, Antonino M, Del Prete V, Panella C, Barone M, Muscatiello N. Polidocanol injection decreases the bleeding rate after colon polypectomy: a propensity score analysis. Gastrointest Endosc. 2015;82(2):350–8.

33. Lenz L, Di Sena V, Nakao FS, Andrade GP, Rohr MR, Ferrari AP Jr. Comparative results of gastric submucosal injection with hydroxypropyl methylcellulose, carboxymethylcellulose and normal saline solution in a porcine model. Arq Gastroenterol. 2010;47(2):184–7.

34. Orsoni P, Berdah S, Verrier C, Caamano A, Sastre B, Boutboul R, Grimaud JC, Picaud R. Colonic perforation due to colonoscopy: a retrospective study of 48 cases. Endoscopy. 1997;29:160–4.

35. Reumkens A, Rondagh EJ, Bakker CM, Winkens B, Masclee AA, Sanduleanu S. Post-colonoscopy complications: a systematic review, time trends, and meta-analysis of population-based studies. Am J Gastroenterol. 2016;111(8):1092–101.

36. Watabe H, Yamaji Y, Okamoto M, Kondo S, Ohta M, Ikenoue T, Kato J, Togo G, Matsumura M, Yoshida H, Kawabe T, Omata M. Risk assessment for delayed hemorrhagic complication of colonic polypectomy: polyp-related factors and patient-related factors. Gastrointest Endosc. 2006;64:73–8.

37. ASGE Standards of Practice Committee, Acosta RD, Abraham NS, Chandrasekhara V, Chathadi KV, Early DS, Eloubeidi MA, Evans JA, Faulx AL, Fisher DA, Fonkalsrud L, Hwang JH, Khashab MA, Lightdale JR, Muthusamy VR, Pasha SF, Saltzman JR, Shaukat A, Shergill AK, Wang A, Cash BD, DeWitt JM. The management of antithrombotic agents for patients undergoing GI endoscopy. Gastrointest Endosc. 2016;83(3):678.

38. Anderloni A, Jovani M, Hassan C, Repici A. Advances, problems, and complications of polypectomy. Clin Exp Gastroenterol. 2014;7:285–96.

39. ASGE Standards of Practice Committee, Fisher DA, Maple JT, Ben-Menachem T, Cash BD, Decker GA, Early DS, Evans JA, Fanelli RD, Fukami N, Hwang JH, Jain R, Jue TL, Khan KM, Malpas PM, Sharaf RN, Shergill AK, Dominitz JA. Complications of colonoscopy. Gastrointest Endosc. 2011;74(4):745–52.

40. Hassan C, Quintero E, Dumonceau JM, Regula J, Brandão C, Chaussade S, Dekker E, Dinis-Ribeiro M, Ferlitsch M, Gimeno-García A, Hazewinkel Y, Jover R, Kalager M, Loberg M, Pox C, Rembacken B, Lieberman D. European Society of Gastrointestinal Endoscopy. Post-polypectomy colonoscopy surveillance: European Society of Gastrointestinal Endoscopy (ESGE) guideline. Endoscopy. 2013;45(10):842–51.

41. Lieberman DA, Rex DK, Winawer SJ, Giardiello FM, Johnson DA, Levin TR. United States multi-society task force on colorectal cancer. Guidelines for colonoscopy surveillance after screening and polypectomy: a consensus update by the US multi-society task force on colorectal cancer. Gastroenterology. 2012;143(3):844–57.

42. Martínez ME, Sampliner R, Marshall JR, Bhattacharyya AK, Reid ME, Alberts DS. Adenoma characteristics as risk factors for recurrence of advanced adenomas. Gastroenterology. 2001;120(5):1077–83.

43. Seo JY, Chun J, Lee C, Hong KS, Im JP, Kim SG, Jung HC, Kim JS. Novel risk stratification for recurrence after endoscopic resection of advanced colorectal adenoma. Gastrointest Endosc. 2015;81(3):655–64.

44. Facciorusso A, Di Maso M, Serviddio G, Vendemiale G, Spada C, Costamagna G, Muscatiello N. Factors associated with recurrence of advanced colorectal adenoma after endoscopic resection. Clin Gastroenterol Hepatol. 2016;14(8):1148–54.

45. Facciorusso A, Di Maso M, Serviddio G, Vendemiale G, Muscatiello N. Development and validation of a risk score for advanced colorectal adenoma recurrence after endoscopic resection. World J Gastroenterol. 2016;22(26):6049–56.

46. Murino A, Hassan C, Repici A. The diminutive colon polyp: biopsy, snare, leave alone? Curr Opin Gastroenterol. 2016;32(1):38–43.

47. Kamiński MF, Hassan C, Bisschops R, Pohl J, Pellisé M, Dekker E, Ignjatovic-Wilson A, Hoffman A, Longcroft-Wheaton G, Heresbach D, Dumonceau JM, East JE. Advanced imaging for detection and differentiation of colorectal neoplasia: European Society of Gastrointestinal Endoscopy (ESGE) guideline. Endoscopy. 2014;46(5):435–49.

48. Ferlitsch M, Moss A, Hassan C, Bhandari P, Dumonceau JM, Paspatis G, Jover R, Langner C, Bronzwaer M, Nalankilli K, Fockens P, Hazzan R, Gralnek IM, Gschwantler M, Waldmann E, Jeschek P, Penz D, Heresbach D, Moons L, Lemmers A, Paraskeva K, Pohl J, Ponchon T, Regula J, Repici A, Rutter MD, Burgess NG, Bourke MJ. Colorectal polypectomy and endoscopic mucosal resection (EMR): European Society of Gastrointestinal Endoscopy (ESGE) clinical guideline. Endoscopy. 2017;49(3):270–97.

49. Sakamoto T, Matsuda T, Nakajima T, Saito Y. Efficacy of endoscopic mucosal resection with circumferential incision for patients with large colorectal tumors. Clin Gastroenterol Hepatol. 2012;10:22–6.

50. Moss A, Bourke MJ, Tran K, Godfrey C, McKay G, Chandra AP, Sharma S. Lesion isolation by circumferential submucosal incision prior to endoscopic mucosal resection (CSIEMR) substantially improves en bloc resection rates for 40-mm colonic lesions. Endoscopy. 2010;42:400–4.

51. Yoshida N, Saito Y, Hirose R, Ogiso K, Inada Y, Yagi N, Naito Y, Otake Y, Nakajima T, Matsuda T, Yanagisawa A, Itoh Y. Endoscopic mucosal resection for middle and large colorectal polyps with a double-loop snare. Digestion. 2014;90:232–9.

52. Binmoeller KF, Weilert F, Shah J, Bhat Y, Kane S. "Underwater" EMR without submucosal injection for large sessile colorectal polyps (with video). Gastrointest Endosc. 2012;75:1086–91.